A CANADIAN HEALTH CARE BLUEPRINT

*Reaching Higher,
Working Smarter, Getting Stronger*

Richard Powlesland

A Canadian Health Care Blueprint
Reaching Higher, Working Smarter, Getting Stronger

Edited by Richard Dionne

Contact: Richard Powlesland
Hwy172021@outlook.com

Print ISBN: 978-1-66789-452-2
ebook ISBN: 978-1-66789-453-9

Printed in the United States of America

A special thanks goes out to Shelley Bradley
for pre-reading the book and making suggestions for improvement.

I especially want to thank my dear wife Rita,
for her patience while I wrote the book.

The book is a tribute to Tommy Douglas. A man who is often recognized for the founding of Canada's Public Health Care System. His vision was to make health care accessible to all. Today we have a publicly funded and managed health care insurance plan. He did want to go further and create a whole new delivery system but it never happened. This book carries on where he left off.

Table Contents

Introduction

Health care is a topic of concern to all Canadians. So, thank you for choosing to read this book. I hope you find it informative. This book was written to inspire you to the possibilities of positive change. The health care topic is not one where solutions to problems come easily. Where to start was the first problem. This is because fixing health care is like pulling on a thread. The more you pull the more it becomes unraveled and will require more work to fix. Each component is dependent on another. This does not mean that change cannot be accomplished, only that any change must take into account many more factors than first come to mind. The book has taken 37 years of experience working as a paramedic in the system to begin to understand the changes that are needed (I am a bit slow, LOL) but there is no doubt that unforeseen circumstances will arise that will necessitate further adaptations.

But why do we need a new health care system? Canadians love our system. Unfortunately, very little of the system is functioning the way it was originally intended to. It is often difficult to find a family physician and then, if you are fortunate enough to have one, there are usually long waits for appointments. Consider also the long waits for the following, ambulance response times, wait times in emergency, consultation appointment with specialists, hospital bed bookings times, having tests completed and sometimes waiting for those results from overworked physicians. All of this takes more time than it should.

Canadians do like the fact that we don't need to worry about pulling out our wallet every time we go to see the doctor or get admitted to the hospital and this is retained in the new proposed system. Canadians like the fact that we get to know our primary health care provider and they get to know us so this will not change and Canadians do like having most of our care provided close to home which will remain. But other things do need to change and one is the family physician/patient relationship. The current system is just not working. Too many problems result in people not receiving care in a timely fashion. Since covid some are not receiving the care at all. Many surgeries in Ontario had to be canceled which may take several years to correct, longer than some people have. Solutions have been found in Manitoba. Cameron MacLean, provides an example, (paraphrasing) the transferring of hip and knee replacement patients, that were delayed because of Covid, will be transferred from Manitoba to out of province [i] Delays also cost money which is explained in the book and governments have their own concerns as costs are rising at a faster pace than they have funding to provide for. This results in changes to the system that have not been able to keep pace with what is needed.

The health care system suggested in the book is called IQSA. It stands for Integrated, Quality, Sustainable, Accessible. The IQSA health care system was designed for Ontario but systems in other provinces and indeed other countries may be able to take advantage of what IQSA has to offer. The IQSA health care system will result in greater efficacy and efficiency and reduce wait times. To address these issues the IQSA system will be based on specialization with new processes that are far more efficient and a new geography of care. The patient, health care provider relationship will be re- envisioned. The infrastructure will adapt to provide the very best. All providers and the system itself will reach higher, work smarter, get stronger and meet the demands.

New plans must address the lapses in the system and do it by being super efficient, accountable and reducing wait times. New ventures designed to boost public funding will help. Some other problems can be addressed by how the health care labour force is engaged. What should be done by whom, when and where. Adding new infrastructure must be limited and instead put what we have to use in new ways. The following statement is paraphrased. A Study indicated that Canadians would like to see one health care system for the country. This was pointed out by Roy Romanow, commissioner of the report, *The Future of Health Care in Canada*.[ii]

This statement was made in 2002 and it has since become apparent that this will not happen. Instead, it will be up to the provinces to figure it out. This book suggests a way for all provinces to manage health care in a new and innovative IQSA way.

Most people feel that when it comes to health care, we have only two choices. Public or private. Neither of these will meet the needs. Both are working with outdated systems that have not kept pace with changes in society. The tools to bring health care into the 21st century is presented in this book and both public and private systems can take advantage of them but it will be up to the people to decide whether more privatization is needed. The IQSA system will update the current system in ways not previously attempted. Privatizing would take less work by the government sector and may be the faster way but is it the best way? If large corporate for-profit clinics take over it may have repercussions beyond health care as corporate profits are shipped out of country leaving less money in circulation here and this could be locked in for a very long time as indicated with the 407 highway that was given a 99-year contract. It does have advantage though in that they can adapt and change much faster than the slower moving public sector. Thomas and Flood, made a good point as they say (paraphrasing) that wait times will not improve through privatizing and instead the system should be modernized.[iii]

In studying health care and other industries, the conclusion drawn is that the best way to go about planning a business and getting the result desired is that first you design the product or end result that you want, then you design the best process you will use to get there and then you built the facilities and train the employees to fit into the system as they are required updating everything as you go along. It works the same no matter what business it is. To do it any other way would result in a complete mismatch of the job requirements and the outcome desired. This has been very difficult to do in health care because some elements are very resistant to change.

CHAPTER 1

The Need for Health Care to Evolve

A lot has been written about health care and what can be done to improve it. And indeed, many things have been done. Pilot projects, a lot of talk and books abound. But that seems to be where it stops. Why does this happen? It may have to do with the way health care has fallen out of synchronization with society. Some of the ideas we see presented may be good on their own, but they are limited. To catch up to the way society is developing, such proposed changes must instead happen on a larger scale. Yes, we currently spend a lot of money and yes, we have large hospitals and employ thousands. But it's not working. By this I mean health care has been done on a small scale. Each physician with their own office, each hospital concentrating mostly on the local population with many small-scale departments to become a general hospital. This narrow focus has dominated the system to date. It also puts limits on health care that needs to be eliminated. But maybe if a new, larger picture is laid out, keeping the best of the current system, folding in some of the pilot projects, adding some new ideas and then you will have a more Integrated Quality Sustainable Accessible (IQSA) system. Imagine it. Not all medical visits have to be to a doctor's office. And not all admissions have to be at a hospital. It can be done. This book is about just such a system and it's called the IQSA system.

Health care has changed immensely since 1966 when the Government of Canada created the Medical Care Act. It made health care public and was a big step forward at the time. The IQSA system enables health care to remain public. It brings health care into the 21st century by updating it to match the way big business functions, especially retail and often manufacturing. Many do so by working 24/7 producing and selling in large quantities. Being a public health care system meant people did not have to go into poverty to pay for essential medical care. People were very happy with it because at the time, they understood it was a first step. But many today are waiting on the necessary second step to take it from an insurance policy to an integrated system.

The ideas for this long awaited second step are about to explode onto the scene like the embers from a smoldering fire blown into a tinder dry forest. Some of these ideas may take hold, but whether health care is private or public, will be up to you because both systems will benefit from the IQSA system presented in this book.

Hopefully we will not lose what Tommy Douglas realized. If you or your child needed any kind of medical attention, the system would be there to pay the physician to look after you, either in the office or the hospital. You along with every other member in your community could go to your family doctor, and they would know you by name and could look after any aliments that you may have. This was a good system and people did like it but with time the costs rose, the system slowed down and became unable to cope with the changes that were happening everywhere. Knowledge in the medical field began to expand rapidly, along with new drugs, treatments, and diagnostic equipment. This might be playing a role in added stress.

A general change in the work/life balance for most in society is flourishing. Few people in any vocation want to spend most of their time at work. This applies to family physicians and their work habits also with fewer working at delivering babies, working in nursing homes or the hospitals. This combined with a higher medical workload due to fewer physicians and an aging population has made things increasingly taxing on both doctors and the elderly.

Keeping pace with these changes by restructuring the way health care is delivered did not happen. At one time a person could make an appointment with the family physician and get in the next day. The physician could make an appointment for a test within a week, and you could see a specialist within two weeks.

But those days are long gone. Just finding a family physician has become difficult. In turn, family physicians tell us that they do not have enough support mechanisms, especially those in rural areas and they feel overworked as do many others. Some of these problems may have started with the physicians but they have now migrated to affect all employees in the health care sector. As all those working in the system become disillusioned as a result, they begin to look elsewhere for employment. Working at improving the system is therefore a must if it is to be there in future. The question, then, becomes what should be done to improve it.

A fresh look at fixing the health care system starts with understanding its history and, society in general. This is because the health care system is not a stand-alone entity. Health care must fit into the way society functions today. This leads to a closer look at how society has evolved in the last century. The health care system did keep pace with society through the 1970s, that is when the last big change to regionalization took place, but since then, it has fallen out of synchronization with the way society functions. Today, anyone can go shopping in huge warehouse-type stores or, if you prefer, you can shop online at any time of day or night that suits you and your schedule best. The array of products and services available for purchase have also grown immensely. People travel much more than they did in the 1940s, 1950s, and 1960s as well (not including Covid lockdowns).

Looking at these factors gives us a starting point. To understand better, a closer look must be taken. It must be understood how society managed to develop these advances. Not all can be attributed to mass manufacturing and technology, but a good portion can be. This is what has raised our standard of living.

Making a product in large quantities allows for a lower selling price thus making it available to more people and increasing profits; this is why it is done. Technology allows for more automation and 24/7 sales. Health care needs to be available to more people. But for the last two decades or so, increasing numbers of people have been unable to get the care they require in a timely fashion. The product or service must be available when it is needed. This is easy to say but not so easy to do. Mass manufacturing is accomplished on an assembly line. It is an essential part of manufacturing. When examined closely, we see that it is creating a smooth flowing process in which each assembly step can be replicated with a predetermined degree of quality, speed, and safety. This is what health care requires. In Henry Ford's time it would be difficult to say that he was automating the process because there were much fewer machines as compared to today. But I would argue that it was the beginning of the automation process because automation is nothing if not a process. The difference at that time was that people had to do most of the assembly work whereas today, a machine might do it.

No matter whether man or machine, neither would work properly if the process had not been carefully developed beforehand. The order and the method had to be perfected. Today with computers, we call it a program or an algorithm. In Henry's time, as it is with health care today, it was a process.

Ford had worked diligently on his own car, designed it, built it, and raced it. When it was ready, he began to experiment with the assembly of his automobile. As he perfected his assembly line (the process), he began to realize additional benefits. Things were moving along much faster than he anticipated. He discovered that the speed of the line was dependent on its slowest point. This is very applicable to health care. He would work diligently at relieving the pressure at that point until things flowed a little more smoothly. At one point, Ford was producing eight cars for every one of his competitors. A smooth health care process would do this. This also meant that he was consuming material at a much higher rate thereby allowing him to purchase in bulk at a much lower price. This would apply to many areas in health care.

Ford also found that because his employees on the assembly line were not required to do a large number of different tasks, they could easily learn to do what was required of them whether it be electrical work or welding, lessening the need for high-cost tradesmen (i.e., electricians and welders whose scope of work was wide). If health care was divided up into a number of smaller tasks, people could possibly be employed with less training. Increasing profits through the savings in the high-cost trades and other measures allowed Ford to pay his average assembly line employee a very good wage, unheard of at the time. He believed that the average worker should be able to afford a car, so he priced his cars equivalent to that of four months of an employee's wages. All health care providers must be paid adequately.

How can we enroll the benefits of our manufactured lifestyle into health care and reap the rewards, such as lower costs, faster service, higher quality, and quicker access for everyone? It is possible, as you will read. In the early days before Henry Ford's Model T the automobile industry consisted of custom engineered, craft-built cars. The process used was sometimes referred to as craft production. It could also be called custom engineering because each part was handmade to fit where it was specifically needed. Often this required filing the part so it would only fit on the vehicle it was intended for. Craft built refers to the fact that all work was completed on one car before starting work on another car. Each craftsman was responsible for many steps in the manufacture of the car. Many companies worked hard at finding ways to eliminate some steps to reduce costs. Occasionally this caused problems for repairs. One automobile manufacturer (not Ford) decided to reduce the time required to build a power train, so they built an engine with the transmission housing permanently attached to the engine, being cast as one unit. The two could not be separated. This saved time, eliminated any filing that might have been required but also made repairs costly. To replace a worn-out transmission required replacing the engine, so selecting the steps in a process, especially in health care, has to be done very carefully. It was not until Ford came along that the automobile assembly line allowed for true mass production. So streamlined was the process that to offer optional paint colours would slow down production and raise costs. So, when choosing your Ford car colour, it was often said you could choose any colour, as long as it was black.

If we were to compare our health care system to the early days of the auto industry, our current system more closely resembles the custom engineered craft-built cars of the past, such as the Pierce-Arrow and Rolls Royce. People loved their custom engineered craft-built cars, but most could not afford them. They were built for the rich or the elite, exclusive in every way. They were not the mass-produced low-cost cars that Ford produced. Ford was inclusive and built for the average person. Those custom engineered craft-built cars worked well on an individual basis, if the individual was in fact rich. They were beautiful cars, often built with meticulous attention to detail and made with the finest materials. Those that purchased them were very happy, regardless of the fact that they were also very, very expensive.

Just like the custom engineered, craft-built car, we liked our health care system in the past but considerably less so now. It is the same one that has been around for a very long time, and has not kept up with changing times. Nothing, stays the same forever, and health care is well on its way to being exclusive, just like the old Locomobile, Pierce - Arrow and Rolls Royce cars. This is most prevalent in the long wait times to gain access for regular Canadians, and the constant threat to privatize as a result. The public system was set up to be inclusive, but to maintain this designation, it will need a major overhaul.

To demonstrate how it got this way we need to closely examine how the system currently works. As an example, when we have an ache or pain, we go to see the family physician. They examine you, may run some tests, diagnose you and prescribe a form of treatment. This process may be different for every patient that this family physician in question treats, including even, those with the same complaint. Some patients may be examined more closely than others or have different tests performed. You could say that each examination and treatment for every patient is custom tailored (engineered) for that individual patient.

Treatment may also vary between physicians and between hospitals with processes very different from each other. Few of us think of this as a system custom made specifically for us, but it is. If you doubt it, the next time you have an ailment, try going to a few different doctors for the same condition. No two treatments will be exactly the same. It can be argued that having different treatments for the same condition in many different people is acceptable because every person is different. However, when treatment of the same patient with the same condition varies from physician to physician, it could be said that other factors are playing a role. Some of the factors may include such things as where the physician received their training and when; or whether the doctor works alone or with others in a team.

This does not mean that there is only one right way. Once all the variable factors are taken into consideration, there may be many effective ways to manage the condition at hand. But is this something that needs to be done in every case? And does the advantage of having so many different approaches outweigh the disadvantages? Ours is a costly system, but one in which the individual does not pay the cost. In a public system it is the society that must bear the cost. This clouds the picture. Patients have no idea of the costs, and less concern. As long as collectively, we can afford it, then this is what we want. As costs rise (or government revenues fall) and funding is reduced, fewer and fewer of us are gaining access to health care in a timely fashion. As a result, we may just start to rethink this strategy.

Our current health care system is similar in ways to the days when all cars were custom engineered and craft built like a Rolls Royce. The Rolls Royce is guaranteed to please the customer too, but it is so costly very few can have the privilege of ownership. So how exactly is our current health care system like one of those custom engineered, craft-built cars? What elements are similar? As it turns out this custom engineered health care system, one in which the physician chooses a treatment plan specifically customized for your needs, like a custom engineered car, is also guaranteed to please and it is also very costly. Just as few people can afford a Rolls Royce, few governments can afford the increasing cost of this customized health care system. So, to control costs there are fewer hospital beds and fewer physicians than required, even though the number of physicians has increased recently the ratio of patients to physicians in the current system is not adequate to meet the need. Today's physicians are not working the long hours of their predecessors, preferring instead a different work/life balance. These factors, among others, have slowed the system down. One topic that is not talked about much is how a slow system cost more. A better understanding is provided by Ernie Stokes that calculates costs under three headings (paraphrased), medical system costs, caregiver costs and patient costs.[iv]

A slow working health care system cost more. Time is money. The patient may lose time from work, may have to redo some tests while waiting for treatment, and delays in treatment generally result in the condition becoming worse which in turn may result in longer patient recovery times and associated cost increases. This may manifest in longer treatment, rehab, medication use, additional time off work, and possibly longer hospital admission time.

Although the current health care system is now much slower than it was in the past, and costs substantially more, it does provide good quality care once access and treatment is gained. Whether this will continue, however, remains to be seen. As the health care knowledge base expands, and more can be done to treat patients' various health concerns, along with increasing demand for service from an expanding (and increasingly elderly) population, the stress and strain to meet the need with the old system becomes irreconcilable. The pressure to work faster in the custom-designed system and to keep up with demand has been building for years and may be resulting in an increase in errors that the medical community sometimes refers to as the adverse effect rate.

In some cases, this may only result in the exclusion of small details. These details may vary greatly from one custom treatment to another and each one of these details may seem insignificant in and of themselves, but some may contribute to the quality of care. As these details are dropped by the wayside, the chance of an adverse effect or omission increases. An example might be a failure to read test results or notify the patient within appropriate time frames. The no news is good news may not be true if the physician did not have time for the chore, or if the physician skipped it altogether, because it was not a remunerated item and therefore not high on the list of "to dos."

This, combined with the need to be knowledgeable in so many more areas than even a decade ago, leaves the family physician in an increasingly difficult position. As a result, we have more physicians specializing. But finding specialists to accept referrals from the family physician can be difficult or the appointment wait times can be very long.

Early Ford cars were different than all others. Most other cars were custom engineered (i.e., parts that only fit one car) and craft-built (assembled one car at a time), that took time to build because the people that worked on them had to be multi-skilled generalists. They were not assigned only one small portion of the work that a Ford assembly line specialist would have been trained to do. The generalists building those beautiful custom engineered, craft-built cars were able to do the work of many specialists but not as quickly as the specialist.

The craft system required that a car sit in one place as the workers moved around it, fitting the parts in place. One worker may have been assigned many jobs that may require many different skills ranging from fitting an engine into place to installing glass and upholstery. It was done this way because the chassis did not move down an assembly line. Work proceeded at a much slower pace because too many workers around the car, would have resulted in crowding, as there was only so much space around the car and crowding would have slowed the process even further.

These generalists were still able to do the job and build beautiful cars, but required more time to look after the many details. Switching from one job to another and picking up where the last one left off took time; the new job often required obtaining different parts, different tools, moving into different positions and understanding how all these parts fit together.

Similar to "multi-skilled generalists, family physicians weighing every treatment option for every condition individually for each patient can take time (custom-designed care). And with medicine able to do so much more for us than in the past, there are many more factors to weigh.

If we want health care to evolve and match or exceed our high standard of living, maybe what we really need would be equivalent to a mass-production Ford with consistently high quality at a lower price. Or, to put it another way, in terms of health care, this would be standard care with a time frame and process clearly defined.

Chapter Highlights

Ford designed and tested the product and then worked at perfecting the process of assembling it until he had everything running as smoothly as he could. This took time but had an immense payoff. Today, nearly everything produced in a modern economy is manufactured on an assembly line. The same attention to process must be done for health care. Engineer the product or service, design the process, built and equip the structure, train the people to meet the needs, and then work at perfecting the process, tweaking as required to eliminate bottlenecks and update regularly. In the end, both process design and health care professionals should complement each other. This is done regularly in manufacturing as the product is redesigned to improve it and retooling takes place sometimes yearly. Then employees are retrained as needed.

Much in our high standard of living society can be attributed to our manufactured lifestyle. A lifestyle defined by the large number of manufactured goods that we consume. The difference is between custom grade and standard grade. The result is a change from purchasing custom made items, built to order, one at a time by generalists, to mass manufactured items, produced hundreds or thousands at a time, by specialists that are defined as people only qualified to do a portion of the work. Standard grade integrated many more products into society, with consistent quality, more efficiently, and affordably, thus making it sustainable Our adoption of the standard grade was generally responsible for our materially wealthy, high-quality, affordable western lifestyle.

CHAPTER 2

Economy of Scale

At some point the health care system will need to change structurally in a way that is different than it has changed to date. Specialization is the future for many reasons. Megan Knoedler notes, (paraphrasing) you tend to get better at something the more you do it plus you tend to get quicker at it and do it safer than others that seldom or rarely do it. [v] Many believe change is only a choice between choosing a public or a private system, but this is not the question at all. Neither system as they are currently designed will meet the needs of the majority. The choice is more about whether we will adopt a standard system, or stay with the fully custom system that we currently have and whether to keep it small scale or expand it as many successful services and companies in our era have done. Whether public or private, both systems could benefit from this new standardized mega-size approach for its economy of scale. Just as in Ford's day, those that could not adapt did not survive. This rule has not changed, no matter how large the institution or industry has become.

The Kodak Company is a good example. It was the largest photography company in the world for a very long time. It *invented* digital photography, but did not pursue it. Kodak knew that if digital photography became popular, it would wipe out Kodachrome, its film business. Kodak needed to make a decision and their people made the wrong choice. Public health care is now facing this type of high-stakes decision. Create new standard treatment regimens performed at specialized Focused Centres of Excellence and other sites or, keep the system functioning the same way for as long as possible, just like Kodak did, and end up facing annihilation.

The need to shift more toward a standard system is mounting. This is because a standard system is far more adaptable to a process and a process can be carefully analyzed to improve many factors, not the least of which is safety. Safety is possibly a bigger issue than many might believe. This is highlighted in an article by James B. Lieber, where he quotes another author's book, Understanding Patient Safety, by Robert M. Wachter, M.D., that I paraphrase. It is difficult to determine the exact number of medical errors in the US but indications are one in ten patients and possibly as high as one in three is associated with a medical error and half could be avoided.[vi]

As the lineup of patients stretches out the door and around the corner, as it did one day in the summer of 2014 at a hospital emergency department in Calgary, we may start to look at other systems. A system that is Integrated, with Quality, is Sustainable and is Accessible (IQSA) is what is needed. A system such as this will allow us to keep our standard of living high in all aspects of our lives. While the current custom system works for those that gain timely access and is praised by those that receive care, it is costly like a Rolls Royce. And the rising cost is unsustainable, resulting in cutbacks which increase the level of deficiency in the custom system. Decades ago, life moved at a much slower pace, and this was when our health care system was designed. Today, everything moves so much faster. I read recently that our current knowledge base is doubling every 10 years. Yet our current system is slow and was not designed for today's needs, but it can be fixed.

Shining a light on the situation may illuminate things that haven't been seen before. Times are changing and consideration must be given to new ways and methods. Understanding and coming to terms with the realization that not all primary care has to be provided by a family physician, and not all admissions have to be made at a hospital, may be the starting point. Focused Centres of Excellence may be the future. What are they? They are part of the IQSA system and are units that *specialize*. They could relieve pressure on hospitals while improving integration.

In the current system, the most common scenario goes like this. The patient has a health concern and goes to their family physician. The family physician does an assessment. Based on the assessment findings and the patient's history, the physician contemplates a number of possible treatment options carefully, weighing all factors and deciding on a plan of treatment. The family physician may find many possible factors that come into play and every patient is treated according to all these factors and their needs. This was a good system, and patients do like it. The complaints about it come in the form of long wait times regarding everything from seeing your family physician to booking a specialist to having scheduled surgery, all delayed due to long waits for admission to a hospital. And then there are government complaints about the cost and public complaints about adverse effects. All these problems and more need to be addressed in order to transform our health care system for the second quarter of the 21st century.

To address the wait times and the costs to society, there are things we can do and indeed they are already being done, but on a very limited basis. Additional money is being funnelled into backlogged surgeries and some patients were sent to other destinations.

If we compare the personalized treatment regimen of every patient and their illness to the early days of automobile manufacture, it could be said that we are in the era of custom engineered craft-built cars. Custom engineered refers to the fact that the parts would only fit the car it was made for. Craft built refers to the fact that cars were built one at a time, with each automobile slowly made to meet the needs of the soon-to-be owner. It is sure to please as long as the individual car purchaser can afford the price of the car.

In the current health care system, the patient receives custom care. Care designed only for one patient. Today, the physician carefully examines each patient. Treatment for the same illness may vary quite a bit from one patient to the next. It varies on the time taken to do an assessment, different types of assessments done, various types of tests done, and numerous types of treatments and drugs prescribed, including the patient's history and current medication list. This can be a good thing or not depending on the results.

A physician once said health care cannot be done cookie-cutter style. What he meant by this is that every patient and their condition is different and must be treated accordingly. This may be true, but it greatly depends on *where you are* in the health care treatment spectrum. Are you normally healthy and receiving your first treatment for a common condition? Or are you on your third visit trying to resolve the same problem? Or are you suffering from a rare form of disease or a chronic condition?

Here's an example. If you went to your family physician with a new ache or pain that is relatively common to the general population, then a standard treatment regimen may work. Treatment for any complaint should normally start off at the least invasive level. Then if the treatment does not work, the patient will return. At this point we must begin to look at other ways of dealing with the problem. Depending on your illness and your family practitioner, they may try numerous treatments, stepping it up a level each time. Maybe ordering more tests and possibly ordering different or stronger drugs or both. A failure to see an improvement or one that is not satisfactory may result in the family physician referring you to a specialist.

Starting any treatment regimen at level one, the least invasive treatment level, is an important first step to working on our problems. As mentioned earlier, providing health care to the patient cannot be done blindly or cookie-cutter style, but depending on the level your treatment is at, it is generally agreed that the least invasive treatment should be the first course of action. The first-contact primary care provider would become the best level to begin IQSA standardization. This approach has worked well for paramedics. Often the first to provide care in an emergency, paramedics do not have the time to consider many different approaches. Their care is standardized through protocols and medical directives. It has proven very effective.

All primary care in first or second contact for an illness or injury should be initially treated according to a standard practice regimen consisting of standard protocols and medical directives. Today's primary treatment regimens can vary widely and are custom designed for each patient. Work is proceeding in some jurisdictions on what is called medical order sets or medical directives. These sets or directives are defined as a grouping of orders used to standardize and expedite the ordering process for a common clinical scenario and may include evidence-based treatment. This is treatment that has been researched and found to have the best outcomes when applied to the condition that it was meant to treat.

Indeed, these standard methods have already been put into practice by some physicians, more so in some jurisdictions than others. There is a trend toward standard care methods that is occurring but on a small single hospital scale as the following statement indicates. The Ontario Hospital Association offers to supply a template for those emergency departments that want to work on standardizing care in their department to increase efficiency, patient flow and patient care.[vii]

This treatment promotes consistency with every patient coming in to the emergency department with the same condition. If applied to primary care, it may result in the patient spending less time with the primary care provider as it would not be a customized the treatment plan. The primary care provider would instead spend less time doing unnecessary assessments, tests, and treatments, especially those that have been proven not to be of general benefit or have a lesser degree of efficacy.

This is a very contentious issue with many physicians because they feel that this is a cookie-cutter approach and does not provide the best care for individual patients. In opposing this approach, they may instead follow a line of treatment more custom engineered for the patient, so to speak. As with the custom engineered automobile, it may prove a slower (and expensive) process with many more options being explored and many more treatments considered. Everything carefully weighed and treatment carefully prescribed according to the patient's needs, the physician's training and experience.

This custom designed treatment results in a high patient satisfaction rating and so it was with custom engineered craft-built automobiles. It also comes with very high costs, just like the custom engineered car, but in this case, it's paid for by society, not by wealthy car buffs.

As a society we pay our physicians very well. They are highly educated and trained and must be able to retain the right to practice their profession in whatever ways they feel is best for their patients. This may include following a standard treatment regimen, possibly evidence based or following care based on their skills, knowledge, experience, and education. Sometimes this may be one and the same, and sometimes not. It would truly be a waste of a lot of good education if physicians were told that they would have to follow the mandated treatment plan called a medical directive (a new standard of care), whether evidence based or not. It would paint them into a corner, so to speak, and I don't believe that this is what society wants. Patients trust their physicians. They want their doctors free to exercise their good judgement in deciding their treatment.

So how can the process be improved? For the purpose of this proposal, evidence-based medical directives would be made standard treatment and would be followed when within the scope of a primary care provider. Specialist care, provided after a consult specialist has been contacted, would only be mandated after a patient's third visit for the same problem when the first and second primary care visits are unsuccessful. In mandating physicians to only follow standard care protocols, there would be no denying that this would be under-utilizing their skills. Canadians have come to expect more of their physicians; and society does benefit by receiving the best value for the high cost involved in training these physicians. So, doctors should not be limited in their abilities or options for treatment.

If we mandate physicians to follow evidence-based medical directives, but society is not ready to accept this from the health care system, then how do we resolve the conundrum and let the system evolve? If family physicians don't work to medical directives or evidence-based care, how would this evolution be accomplished? A change such as this might work better if introduced at the front lines. And maybe, as we go along, a closer look at health care provider roles will yield some more answers.

On closer examination, some of the duties of a family physician could be divided up. This has already been done in some areas as we've seen with the introduction of midwives that have taken over deliveries for many family physicians. Ontario has opened nurse practitioner-led clinics in Ontario and they provide comprehensive care along with a team-based approach that may include a registered nurse, a dietitian, a social worker, and a consulting doctor. Nurse practitioner clinics are working well. When introduced they required some family physician contact. One reason was because they were not able to prescribe narcotics but that was when they were considered a new model of care and this has since changed.[viii]

Paramedics are now providing community care that has cut back the number of patients needing to go to the emergency department.

As the knowledge base grows in any one field, society divides up the workload and creates specialists to manage and make sense of all this incoming information. This might be similar to the approach that could be used by paramedics at **primary** emergency care centres. Few fields have increased their knowledge base like the field of medicine. Today the field of medicine has many thousands of known diseases and twice as many drugs approved for use. It is very difficult for a general practitioner, family physician, emergency physician or anyone for that matter, to know all there is to know in every medical or surgical field, as these areas are very large and expansive indeed.

Even the information well known today may very well become quickly outdated. These high-knowledge expectations place a great deal of stress on today's physicians. This was highlighted one day on a health care radio program on CBC radio, hosted by Dr. Brian Goldman. (paraphrased) Here, an ER physician talked about all the questions medical students had for him, many of which he could not answer. When he explained that they would need to direct some of their questions to specialists, the students seemed surprised as they expected him to have the answers.[ix] The explosion of new medical information has made the ability to know all or what is best 100% of the time impossible; and it is time to lessen this expectation, and in turn, lessen the stress levels of physicians.

There are few solutions to this problem other than western societies tried and true answer, divide up the workload and create specialists. The two main remaining duties of a family physician are their office duties and emergency care.in a few cases but the government is staffing ERs with emergency physicians whenever possible.

As it turns out, changes to the way that family (general) practitioners work has been occurring gradually for some time. Fewer doctors are choosing to practice in rural and remote areas, and fewer doctors want to go out in an ambulance. Indications are that 8% of physicians were located in rural areas and 92% were concentrated in urban areas. Our health care system started adapting to these changes in the 1960s and 1970s. It was then the modern type of nurse practitioners (NPs) and paramedics entered the health care scene. Unfortunately, it took a long time for society to "fully" utilize these highly trained and knowledgeable professionals by allowing them to practice what they learned in urban settings in Ontario for nurse practitioners, and in primary health care for paramedics in some jurisdictions. As the internet becomes a more integral part of health care, even more nurse practitioners and paramedics will be utilized. If we continue with this shift these two professions, specialists in their own right, may take over the bulk of primary care and primary emergency care. Primary emergency care is the same as urgent care (emergency care that does not require a hospital stay) with two distinct differences: It is care provided by paramedics, not physicians, and it is open 24/7.

Nurse practitioners cannot do all that a family physician was trained to do, but they can manage the work done in the office. Family physicians were taught at one time to provide many more services such as delivering babies, emergency department work, operating room work and setting fractures, although today very few family physicians work in areas outside the office. Primary care and primary emergency care may make a considerable change to the conditions in emergency departments but they may need to have longer hours. Health Sciences North (the Sudbury Hospital) CEO, Dominic Giroux, discovered that the reason many patients, (half of those coming to the emergency department), do so because of difficulty in getting in to see their family physician in a timely manner.[x]

Paramedics are specialists also, and they could take over primary emergency care. This type of work was once done by family physicians in their office or at a hospital. It was work where the patient did not require admission. (i.e.: setting a fractured arm) If paramedics provide primary emergency care, it would be replacing only a portion of the family physician's training. It would entail such things as suturing, setting and casting simple fractures prior to assessment by a specialist. Today this type of care may be carried out at an urgent care centre by physicians. Today, paramedic care concentrates on pre-hospital emergency care but is gradually shifting to include more out-of-hospital and community care. This means they are also focusing on patients that are treated to the degree that transport to a hospital may no longer be required or they check on the well-being of an aging population, or those patients that use emergency departments frequently. Creating PECC 's would circumvent the need for some patients to go to the emergency department.

Currently we have two levels of community paramedics that provide care to patients at home. ACP community paramedics (advanced-care paramedics) and PCP community paramedics (primary care paramedics), both provide additional home care for patients, with ACP community care paramedics providing additional care for chronic COPD, CHF, and diabetics.

If paramedics and nurse practitioners take over the bulk of work in these two areas, what would become of our highly regarded family physicians? As in any field, as the knowledge base expands and becomes too much for any one profession, specialists are created to divide up the huge inflow of information and make sense of it. This is what has been done in the past and it is still societies solution today. As broad-based training and the variety of work of the family physician is divided up, family physicians will need additional training to become specialists. This would be the biggest challenge in health care in a century, and it is not a recommendation taken lightly. The stress that family physicians are under may stem from many different reasons, but not having enough supports might be one. Alex McKeen discovered fewer medical students are choosing to become family physicians. It may also be explained as having something to do with the following statement. (paraphrased) Family physicians have a huge and growing workload and medical students see this during their schooling and are deciding its not for them.[xi] Some might say that this would mean a degradation of the health care system, but I believe it would be a giant step forward in the IQSA system. It will assure that care can be provided by specialists for everyone in the new IQSA Health Care System.

Providing care at all times day or night when the patient requires it will in itself bring about better results. Don't get me wrong. The current system does the best it can to provide care as quickly as possible, but not all get the care they need, at the time they need it, and having to wait until after the weekend or even the next day or longer can shorten lives, increase pain and suffering, and cost the health care system more. A service as important as health care should not be an outlier. Service 24/7 would be in keeping with the way society functions today. People can go shopping any time of the day or night 7 days a week and people travel at all hours. The red-eye fights are an example of this. Faster service has always been a goal underlying our current health care system, but it has not worked out that way. Rural areas have always been understaffed and now urban areas have long wait lists. Problems are multiplying as public services struggle with increasing demand and less funding and staff.

To accomplish this giant step, we will need to have a plan to provide the primary care that family physicians were providing. What types of work are most family physicians practicing? Most have already given up obstetrics and few do any work in the operating room or the emergency department. There are two distinct areas of practice for a family physician, primary care in the office, and some provide hospital or clinic and walk-in care. Some family physicians have taken on more responsibilities, but most have not.

As mentioned, and which bears repeating: there are two groups of health professionals that are well suited to take over primary care and primary emergency care responsibilities. Both paramedics and nurse practitioners have been around for a very long time. Nurse practitioners first came on the scene in the 1960s and paramedics in the 1970s. Both have seen major changes in their scope of practice. They are primed to manage the change to evidence-based medical directives. In this group of health care professionals, nurse practitioners would provide primary care in the office and they have in fact already started doing so. Paramedics, on the other hand, would provide primary emergency care. At one time, in the 1970's and early 1980's while I was at work, at one of our ambulance stations. A patient, on occasion, would show up at the door requesting medical care. One case had a laceration and needed a dressing. After doing that we made arrangements to transport the patient to hospital. To our surprise the patient steadfastly refused, so we advised him to see his family physician later at which point he left. It happened a few more times to me but management made efforts to prevent it from happening and eventually patients stopped coming to the door of the ambulance station. The fact it happened more than once was when I realized the untapped potential. Other jurisdictions (Nova Scotia) managed the situation differently as demonstrated by Kristopher Morrison in the following statement (paraphrased) Long waits for family doctors' appointments and regular emergency department closures forced a new way of doing things and they created emergency rooms without doctors. [xii] They were staffed by nurses and paramedics.

Primary emergency care is defined as emergency care that does not require admission to a hospital (i.e., suturing small lacerations). Primary emergency care would become a branch of emergency care. Anytime that a patient has a problem that is beyond the health care providers' scope of practice, a referral will be made. This referral may be to the emergency department physician or others depending on the urgency. Both paramedics and nurse practitioners have been doing this for a long while, but now with this plan, they will be going mainstream. Of course, the time frame for this shift in care would be slow. As more family physicians and medical students choose a specialty, then more nurse practitioners and paramedics would be employed.

In the case of paramedics, they already treat according to standard protocols and medical directives. The transition to primary emergency care would see the use of evidence-based care used in medical directives developed for every condition that would be treated at a primary emergency care centre. Paramedics are not educated to the degree that a physician is, and they are not remunerated like a physician. This has not prevented their treatment regimens from providing excellent results. Extending their capabilities to primary emergency care centres would allow for some diversion from the hospital emergency department and speed up service for all those patients that do not require admission.

If we look back at what Ford did, he created a system, moreover, a process. He managed to speed up the process and lower the costs all the while maintaining quality. He paid well but he did not hire those trained in the trades (licensed electricians, welders, etc.). Rather he limited the scope of the job for the men on the line to the degree that they were able to replicate the results that would have been equally obtained by the licensed trades person for that given application. In other words, an assembly line employee with fine skills training in a limited capacity or specialty, was able to replicate the quality of the specialized trades in a limited capacity, without the education, training or multiple skills of the trade's professional people. This was done by having line workers adhere to a strict process. One that did not require the full scope of training of a licensed trades person (e.g., say that of a licensed electrician) but could do only a portion of the work. If a wider scope of specialized work was required, Ford could always hire a licensed trades person, which he did on occasion. This represented a huge cash saving for Ford who was then able to pay his employees better and pass on savings to the purchaser.

Chapter Highlights

Primary health care is provided by a customized care system that must shift to a mainstream standard/custom system. All standard care will be evidence based. Many will have you believe that the only choice for health care is either public or private, but this is not the question at all. Neither of those will meet our needs. The question should be phrased instead as: will it be a fully custom system which is what we have now in both public and private care, or will we transition to a new system which is a blend of custom and standard care?

CHAPTER 3

The All-Specialists Health Care System

Exciting times are ahead as we transform into the world's best health care system. That is the IQSA system. All specialists working in a system designed for them will bring the finest care to all patients, at all times, on budget, non-stop. The restructuring of health care into the IQSA health care system will take time and will not be easy, but it can be done. We must remember it was not easy to bring about a public health care system in Canada and the IQSA system will require as much effort as in the past.

If the change to non-physician primary care providers takes place, as it has in some jurisdictions already (although not exclusively), and family physicians are moved forward to become specialists, it will be a fundamental transition that will put Canada at the forefront of health care, and truly, a world leader. The IQSA system is a long-range goal. The 10 to 15 years that it may take to implement would mean that no new family physicians would be trained and those retiring, leaving or becoming specialists, would not be replaced. The normal attrition/retirement rate of family physicians along with those upgrading will allow for a gradual shift to an all-specialists system.

The question becomes, how is the situation managed if the **primary care** specialists (registered nurse practitioners) or the **primary emergency care** specialists (paramedics), have a problem beyond their scope of practice? Currently, they may contact a family physician or a specialist. If the future has fewer or no family physicians, the system will be dependent on specialists, but some specialists are already in short supply. So how do we fix this problem? The current shortage of specialists will be remedied by training more family physicians to become specialists.

Paramedics and nurse practitioners have been expanding their knowledge base for years, enabling them to do more. Some places have decided to put paramedics to work in new ways in a clinical setting. Nova Scotia is not the only place where paramedics work in clinics or emergency departments. Martin Schuldaus in an article wrote (paraphrasing) Alberta is doing this also where in 2010 a clinic in northern Alberta provides both clinical and emergency care by paramedics and all care is within their scope of practice. [xiii] As these front-line professionals climb the ladder of knowledge, those on the rungs above will also reach higher. What does this mean? It means that as nurses and paramedics at the front line develop into new types of specialists and gain a specific portion of the knowledge that the general/family physician has, they will become the "go to" for those areas of care where they specialize. In one controversial pilot project in the UK, Sophie Borland indicates (paraphrased) paramedics and will carry out home visits, prescribe drugs and do routine appointments with training similar to a GP. They are doing this because of a shortage of GP's but it is noted that prescribing drugs is only after proper training to maintain safety. [xiv] In the IQSA system the physicians that were doing this work will reach higher and become specialists also. All of this will make a tremendous difference to the system and will alleviate the system of the shortage of specialists.

With all family physicians reaching higher and becoming specialists, it eliminates the need to increase the length of time required for the family physician training program. Currently, family physicians are under increasing pressure to expand their knowledge base, but this poses a problem. How long should the family physician training program be? Is it reasonable to extend the length of the program so that family physicians are able to cover more of the expanding knowledge base?

Strange as this may sound, in the United States they now have an accelerated medical school program reducing the general practitioner education time frame from four to three years. The NYU Grossman School of Medicine in Manhattan is one of these schools. The reason given for this is a shortage of GPs and what is referred to as the cost/benefit ratio. The US has determined that fewer applicants are applying for general practitioner programs because the general practitioner (GP) earns less than a specialist. This results in student loan repayment taking longer. This longer time frame, referred to as the cost/benefit ratio, makes the GP degree much less appealing. A three-year medical degree may attract more students to the general (family) physician program, but it does nothing to lessen the stress caused by increased general knowledge expectations as the following statement explains where Dyrbye, Liselotte N. MD; Thomas, MathewR.MD; Shanafelt, Tait D. MD (paraphrased) Psychological distress starts in med school and may be leading to depression but there is insufficient information to draw firm conclusions. [xv] In an age when the knowledge base is expanding quickly, to reduce the time for education is to expand the knowledge gap. It would better benefit society if family physicians upgraded their training to specialist levels and the current family physician workload was divided up and assigned to other specialists.

Looking at the problem from another perspective might provide insight into the US dilemma. The medical field knowledge base is expanding rapidly. Rather than extending or shortening GP training time, it might be better to take a system approach and upgrade the general/family physician's knowledge base through additional training so they become specialists. This then requires others to increase their knowledge base, raising all to a higher level. This is preferable to going in reverse.

If this were to happen, how can the public system afford to train so many specialists? The cost of training more family physicians to become specialists would be much less costly than training specialists from scratch, offset because of the training they already have. They are qualified physicians, the additional cost of specializing, depending on the specialty they choose will vary. Having more specialists will increase system costs but increased efficiency will offset this cost if the care they provide is optimized. The system must be designed so that specialists do only that work which only they have the expertise to do. An example of this is a hospital in Winnipeg where the orthopedic surgeon comes into the OR to replace a knee only after the physician assistant has prepared the patient by opening the site. The surgeon then replaces the knee and proceeds to the next patient while the physician assistant returns to close the site.

The system needs more physician specialists. Adding more physician specialists through additional training for our family physicians means that the primary care system will not have family physicians. The funding once used to support family physicians may now be transferred between the cost of providing primary care replacements and providing additional physician specialists. Now I know that you are probably thinking, what will all these specialists do? Some will be researchers, and some will be system process developers, but the majority will be additional system specialists to provide the best care possible. This is because care will be provided in a new and exciting way. This is the IQSA system, focused and specialized, working 24/7 for you, the patient.

The shift to more specialists and fewer family physicians began many decades ago. Specialists would have outnumbered family physicians by now but the provincial government, fearing too many people were without a primary care provider, began to increase medical school enrollment with an emphasis on family physicians. Municipalities also stepped in to provide incentives to attract family physicians. These steps helped increase the number of family physicians, but some patients are still without a family doctor and primary care hours are still limited, meaning *not* 24/7.

The all-specialist system has many advantages. Here are but a few:

1. The health care system will be able to fill in the shortage of specialists.

2. It may divide up the incoming information among more specialists and more sub-specialists.

3. It will allow for quicker referrals.

4. It will assist in the problem of trying to determine health-related human resource allocation. Some specialists will be both family physician and specialist as they await an opening for a full-time specialist.

5. Family physicians can continue to practice as they learn a specialty, allowing more time for the system to adjust as change takes place.

6. Those patients requiring longer recovery periods may spend time at their local tertiary care hospital, formerly the community general hospital where the patient will continue to be cared for virtually by the Focused Specialist. (FS)

Currently, it is difficult determining how many specialists in any given field may be needed. Sometimes too many have been trained and sometimes there are not enough. One way to lessen this problem is by having physicians run a dual practice. They would be both family physician and specialist. If more specialists in a given field were needed, those in a dual practice would be given the opportunity to work full time in their specialty. This dual practice physician position could be a technique used primarily during the transition to a fully specialist system, but it may continue to a lesser extent to assure the system has the specialists available when required.

Some other jurisdictions experienced shortages of family physicians long before us. In some big cities such as Los Angeles, specialists began doing primary care but maintained their specialist qualifications. As patients came to them, they were treated as required, either through the field of primary care, or, if the patient's problem fell within the physician's specialty, then the same physician would provide that care. If it happened that the patient needed specialist care in another field, they would be referred. Remuneration could be consistent with the type of care provided.

The IQSA operating system shift to an all-specialist medical system is going to produce many more specialists than the current system has. As you read through this book, you will see how these additional specialists will be put to work and how it will be done in such a way as to minimize additional costs to the system.

Over time, the way that family physicians practice has changed. Today, it is much different than in the 1940s, 1950s, and 1960s. In those bygone days, family physicians often delivered babies, did house calls, and would when required, go into the operating room and remove an appendix; they would routinely work in the emergency room, and they would often set fractured bones and do suturing in their office or at the hospital.

Today, just about the only thing that some family physicians will do outside their office is work the emergency department; and even this is changing as the government is requiring emergency departments to be staffed by emergency specialists. Midwives have taken over the uncomplicated deliveries family physicians once did, and obstetrician specialists do the rest. General surgeons and specialists now do all operating room work, including the appendix removal once done by family physicians. Most fractured bones are set in temporary casts by orthopedic technicians and are then referred to orthopedic specialists. House calls may occasionally still be done by a few family physicians, but it is mostly now done by nurses, paramedics, and personal support workers, depending on the patients' condition.

As it turns out, nurse practitioners are already providing care for patients in office settings. Ontario has established nurse practitioner-led clinics and as was mentioned previously, in Nova Scotia, paramedics with nurses staffed the emergency department at night during a physician shortage. In the future, paramedics could fill in for family physicians by providing only a portion of the work they did and that is *primary* emergency care. This is the type of emergency care that does not require hospital admission.

This transition should be spread out slowly over 15 years or less. Some new physician specialists may continue to act in dual mode as family physician/specialist, but the majority will not. To fill the gap in primary health care with the departure of family physicians, nurse practitioners and paramedics will step forward. Each specialized to provide a portion of what the family physician provided. The nurse practitioner will be providing all care that was provided by the family physician in the office, and the paramedic will provide primary emergency care currently mostly provided in hospital emergency departments and sometimes at urgent care centres. These two services may then increase service to 24/7. Both groups, backed up by greatly increased access to specialists, and indeed mandated through the H2C in some cases. All of this is made possible by new technology such as video conferencing.

This major change in health care to an all-specialist health care system would have a number of benefits. It would increase safety, reduce diagnostic errors, improve treatment plans, build focused excellence and, tied in with other changes, it would increase efficiency and efficacy. Special consideration will be given to family practitioners to receive additional training. By this I mean they may continue to work as family practitioners but will train toward specialization. During the transition they may maintain part-time family practice if they prefer, and they may do this in future if they desire, becoming a dual family practitioner/specialist, but this may result in frequent travel to the nearest Focused Centre of Excellence for that specialty. The IQSA RR may assist with incentive funding for those physicians training in the specialty that their IQSA RR will specialize in.

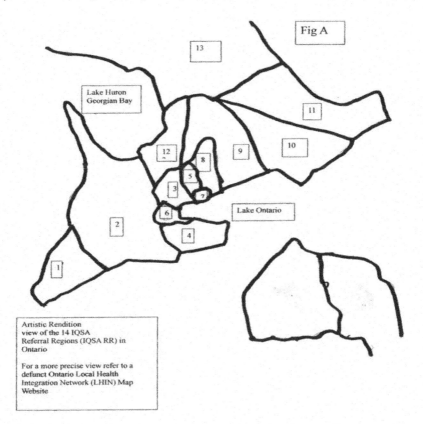

Having a specialist provide primary care is nothing new. Specialists are general practitioners that have received additional training in a specialty. In the 1980s Ontario changed the title "general practitioner" to "family physician" and decided it would not let specialists use the term family physician as a fall back, but specialists are actually qualified to provide primary care if required. This, however, may not be the best use of these highly trained specialists, so while having a specialist provide primary care may work, after the transition to the all-specialist system, other arrangements for the bulk of primary care should be made. This would involve training nurse practitioners and paramedics to provide the care normally provided by the family physician.

Chapter Highlights

The new health care system will consist of all specialists. All family physicians will train to become specialists, providing the best care for everyone day or night 24 hours a day. Others already in the system will provide the majority of services that they provided, but will have new supports built into the system.

CHAPTER 4

Focused Centres of Excellence

The future will be terrific. The IQSA Health Care System will be composed of all specialists. The next step will be to determine how the specialists will work. This will play a major role in how the health care system functions and how all patients benefit. The proposed changes will have everyone working at their best, providing the finest care possible. Physician specialists will be working at new centres called "Focused Centres of Excellence." These centres will be equally distributed among the IQSA RRs throughout the province.

The Focused Centres of Excellence will become the new standard benefiting all patients. Matching the patient and the specialist to the facility specifically designed for them and their need. This will be advantageous for both. The best of care provided within a reasonable time frame with the goal a three-week maximum wait for a Focused Centre of Excellence admission and a one day wait for a primary care appointment.

It was recognized a long time ago that specialization provides the best care when admission to a hospital was required and that is why we have physician specialists. Building on this by transforming to a full specialist system will provide the best care possible for everyone. Advancing one more step by creating **Focused** Centres of Excellence that operate with physician specialists onsite 24/7 will mean that the best care is provided any time of day, another major step toward the world's best health care system.

The idea behind this is to provide the very best care non-stop. Specialists can provide this care in ways others cannot and with the new IQSA health care system, they are able to provide it as quickly as possible. Emergency patients always receive priority and although this is the case in the current system, many patients do not receive that care as soon as desired. Sometimes staff required for specific procedures are absent, may be off for the night or on vacation. This intermittent need to call in staff results in delays. Sometimes those called in are not specialized in the necessary procedure which may slow things down.

All patients at Focused Centres of Excellence will receive care at the time they need it in a specialized unit for the type of care they require. This will present huge health benefits for patients. A patient's stay there will be a maximum of four days. All patients will receive prompt specialist care. Most through the standard care program. That is the evidence-based care program designed for the best possible result and may reduce treatment time. In many cases, the patient may be discharged home after Focused Centre of Excellence care but for some, more time to recover may be needed, and they may receive home care or be transferred to a tertiary care hospital to allow for additional recuperation, but this need is decreasing for some patients as the following statement by Haute Autorite de Sante indicates (Paraphrased) Day Surgeries, those that do not require a bed or an overnight stay, may be in for an increase if as they say admitting patients for the shortest amount of time may be possible in eight out of ten surgeries.[xvi] The four days allotted for Focused Centres of Excellence may work well for surgery. The medical cases may vary. They give examples of some types of surgery suited to day surgery, such as routine and common procedures including surgery for cataracts, hernia, varicose veins and hand conditions. Some countries include complex surgery such as, gall bladder, gastro-oesophageal reflux, shoulder, thyroid and obesity.

The Focused Centre of Excellence approach would eliminate expensive equipment sitting idle, real estate going unused, utility bills accumulating without a purpose, health providers not utilized to the full extent of their training, and patients' tests and treatments becoming outdated or put on hold, all of which occur in today's facilities where all staff do not work 24/7 or are not kept up to date on the latest advances.

The Kensington Eye Institute in Toronto is a day surgery clinic (no overnight stay) which specializes in cataract and other types of eye surgery has proven that it is possible to treat many more patients in less time at lower cost. It was a major step forward in its day, highly specialized and working well but taking it one more step to a 24/7 service will enhance it even further. This approach, when applicable, will be applied to all Focused Centres of Excellence in the IQSA system

The new Focused Centres of Excellence would be very large, specialized units serving the whole province and possibly beyond. There would be three sizes of focused units: a minimum 200-bed unit, a 300-bed unit, and a maximum 400-bed unit. The units would be distributed evenly among all IQSA RR coverage areas. By this I mean there would be three Focused Centres of Excellence for each IQSA RR coverage area, and they may or may not be all the same size. Anything under a 200-bed unit could not be made economically efficient enough to meet the IQSA standard. Over 400 beds the unit becomes harder to manage and thus loses efficiency. Due to their size, there is the possibility of these large units developing sub-specialties within the unit further improving care. The IQSA system will make us world leaders. With 24/7 operation, these giant-size units will create an efficient, quality health care system with better outcomes at lower cost per capita, meeting the needs now and well into the future. Creating focused units will present opportunity for widespread process improvement and lower supply chain costs utilizing bulk purchasing, while going super-size will lower the number of units required for treatment of a condition and result in more efficient use of equipment and time.

The internet has made 24/7 service a reality in many business sectors. People can shop online anytime. Goods are shipped day and night. Society is changing and health care needs to change with the times. That's why 24/7 utilization 365 days a year will benefit everyone. Better management of the workforce is essential to improve the system. It is understood that in an emergency, time is of the essence. Many a patient have had heart attacks or some other condition when the specialist and their team was not at the hospital and had to be called in. This takes time. Sometimes procedures are delayed because they fall on the weekend, or in the middle of vacation time. Sometimes less experienced or unlikely candidates are recruited to fill in. The longer the patient waits for care the more damage that is done and the longer it takes to return to health. This is not just true in an emergency, but in nearly every condition that a patient may have. Can you imagine the benefits to society in terms of lost work time alone, and how this could be reduced if care could be provided sooner. John Dujay writes (paraphrased) Lost productivity and wages in Canada has amounted to almost 2.1 billion because of long waits for medical treatment and surgery.[xvii]

Using a Focused Centre of Excellence approach may eliminate a problem that plagues our current system. In the beginning of my paramedic career, I worked on an ambulance that was stationed at a small-town hospital. It was an old hospital built by the town's main employer in a time before public health care. The hospital wanted to modernize, to build a new delivery room, nursery, and operating room, but these additions were not feasible.

Instead, plans for a new hospital were made. After many years of planning and fundraising a new hospital was built. It was beautiful with its new delivery room, nursery, and operating room. Unfortunately, the physicians that were to provide these services retired before the new units were completed. The small hospital worked hard to recruit an obstetrician and a surgeon, but to no avail. Years later (approximately 10), they gave up trying and renovated the unused space into patient rooms.

Problems with recruitment that lead to this type of waste should be greatly minimized at Focused Centres of Excellence. A supportive work environment with many other "same type" specialists working together in dedicated surgical and medical units with specialized equipment, fast-paced progressive treatment, and dedicated processes will all be factors easing problematic recruitment and turnover rates. And this must be one of many priorities as human resource problems in health care are increasing. In Ontario, the ministry does more than it did in the past assisting towns with physician recruitment or locums (staff that fill in for vacations, etc.) to help staff emergency departments. However, staffing problems are now involving more than just physicians. Many other health care providers are now in short supply in towns where it was never a problem. High workload and the availability of mostly part-time employment and small pay increases during high inflation may be part of the problem. Further study is needed but efforts should be made at curtailing this trend.

The IQSA system presents possible answers to some of these variables in ways not attempted before. With fewer units there would be less competition at recruitment drives. The IQSA system will bring stability and less stress for all staff, possibly further easing recruitment problems.

A well-designed system, both physical and operational, will attract specialists and other health care providers to it and retention will be easier. Once a good process has been devised the system will require regular updates to keep it current. Good design and operational processes are essential to keeping costs down and for patient efficacy. In the last couple of decades or so there has been a mismatch between facilities and professionals able to do the work. It varies from having the staff but not the facilities to complete the work, to there being adequate facilities and not enough staff. Mismatches such as these may always be present to some degree, brought about on purpose but not always. Larger swings may have become notable. Sometimes these miscalculations result in needless expense such as when many more operating rooms are built than are needed, or can be staffed. The change to Focused Centres of Excellence will alleviate many of these issues by narrowing down the scope of local management concerns to one, two or three types of focused units within the IQSA RR, rather than the wide range of care a hospital provides today. Having to manage too many factors within a wide range of health care concerns tends to pull management's attention in many directions at the same time and may lead to miscalculations. To some degree, tertiary care may still be confronted with providing care for many types of injury or illness but the patients are virtually cared for by specialists from other sites.

With an all-specialist system and an expanding knowledge base, care will improve but only if that knowledge is put to work to optimize care and gain the most health benefit for the greatest number of patients at the best price. This in turn will depend on how the skills and knowledge of the professionals are utilized or, you could say, by determining how best to do the work required.

Becoming larger, as the Focused Centres of Excellence are, is following through with practices put into motion years ago in some jurisdictions. In the US many hospitals grew into large corporations encompassing many hospital sites as pointed out in the following article by Kenneth L. Davis (paraphrased) Many were worried when hospital mergers became the thing to do decades ago. They assumed it would decrease competition and raise costs but it didn't happen as expected and now offers the possibility of more efficiency and higher quality [xviii]

The process change to all Focused Centres of Excellence will provide that new working environment. It will be better for patients but will also rejuvenate all care providers knowing that they can and will meet the needs of patients in ways they never could before and allow them to be their best. Centres of excellence are already in existence. **Focused** Centres of Excellence are new. The primary difference is these new units are very large, serve the entire province and possibly beyond, and provide care with specialists onsite 24/7. They are units of specialized care. In some cases, they may be the only occupant in what was once a general hospital.

All Focused Centres of Excellence will care for hundreds of people at the same time, thousands over a year. Each focused unit will have its own ICU section. While the prime prerequisite for opening a Focused Centre of Excellence will be the ability to function with specialists onsite 24/7. Faster service, lower cost, greater output, and higher quality will all add up to a superior Canadian system, the IQSA health system, best in the world.

Although suggestions have been made, it is beyond the scope of this book to determine the number of focused units in any one category, the size of the various categories of care, the location of the Focused Centres of Excellence within an IQSA RR or the type of care they provide within the IQSA RR. More study and collaboration would be required to determine these elements.

The following is for demonstration purposes, just to give you an idea of what the system could look like if the Focused Centres of Excellence were divided equally among the IQSA RR. The decision on the services that each IQSA RR delivers will be decided among the IQSA RRs, lead hospitals, and the Ministry of Health and Long-Term Care with emphasis on whenever possible, working with each IQSA RR to specialize in one, two or three categories of care within three Focused Centres of Excellence.

All care is based on a Focused Centre of Excellence maximum stay of four days with a ratio of one specialist there caring for five in-patients and video conferencing with up to five more per day. These additional five patients could be located at a tertiary care hospital, a primary care centre, a primary emergency care centre or a hospital emergency department or other locations to be determined. So, while this is the goal, the number of patients seen per day would vary. Some patients may require more time while some less.

Examples of categories of care provided by Focused Centres of Excellence:

For information on current statistics such as the number of hospitals in Ontario or the number of beds please google Ontario Hospital Association, OHA Fact Sheet on Hospital Capacity. For information on current number of specialists in Ontario please go to the Ontario Medical Association website OMA website under What We Do and OMA factsheet for the number of practicing physicians

1 Gastroenterology	2 Allergy & Immunology
3 Cardiology	4 Trauma
5 Neurology	6 Ophthalmology
7 Ear Nose & Throat	8 Infectious Diseases
9 Psychiatry & Mental Health	10 Geriatrics
11 Orthopedics	12 Obstetrics
13 Gynecology	14 Diabetes
15 Endocrinology	16 Plastic Surgery & Dermatology
17 Urology	18 Oncology
19 Pulmonology	20 Pediatrics
21 Rheumatology	22 Nephrology
23 Internal Medicine	

In total there are 42 Focused Centres of Excellence providing 23 categories (types) of care. In the beginning each IQSA RR would have one Focused Centre of Excellence of each size, one 200-, one 300-, and one 400-bed unit. During development one size may be exchanged if another IQSA RR can be found to do a swap with. The categories of care that are chosen for each IQSA RR would be determined in consultation with the

IQSA RR, the hospital that provides the service, and the Ministry of Health and Long-Term Care.

All recommendations are based on a focused unit maximum stay of four days. The following example will indicate: the number of patients to be cared for at Focused Centres of Excellence.

The following calculations are only one example of the many possibilities:

1. The Number of Patients to Receive Care at Focused Centres of Excellence in One Year

Based on one treatment taking four days

For 14 - 400 bed units

7.5 treatments per bed every 30 days x 400 beds per unit = 3000 treatments every 30 days

3000 treatments every 30 days x 12 months = 36,000 per year x 14 units = 504,000 treatments per year

For 14-300 bed unit

7.5 treatments per bed every 30 days x 300 beds per unit = 2,250 treatments every 30 days

2,250 treatments every 30 days x 12 months = 27,000 per year x 14 units = 378,000 treatments per year

For 14-200 bed units

7.5 treatments per bed every 30 days x 200 beds per unit = 1,500 treated every 30 days

1,500 treatments every 30 days x 12 months = 18,000 per year x 14 units = 252,000 treatments per year

Total number of patients treated at all Focused Centres of Excellence

504,000 + 378,000 + 252,000 = 1,134,000 patients treated per year.

This number of patients capable of being treated per year at Focused Centres of Excellence may leave room to innovate.

Tertiary care hospitals will consist of the beds that remain after all Focused Centres of Excellence bed requirements have been met. The overall number of beds in the system will not change.

2. The Total Number of Focused Centres of Excellence Beds

Number of Beds in IQSA Focused centres of excellence

The number of beds 400 x 14 units = 5,600

The number of beds 300 x 14 units= 4,200

The number of beds 200 x 14 units = 2,800

Total 12,600 beds

The total number of Focused Centres of Excellence Beds = 12,600

3. The Number of Specialist Physicians Required for All Focused Centres of Excellence

Note: based on one physician caring for five focused in-patients per day; if working 12 hours per day or 8 hours per day

For one 400-bed focused unit:

400 divided by 5 = 80 physicians x 14 focused units
= 1,120 physicians at

12-hour shifts per day 1,120 x 2 = 2,240

8-hour shifts per day1,120 x 3 = 3,360

For one 300-bed focused unit:

300 divided by five = 60 physicians x 14 focused units
= 840 physicians at

12-hour shifts per day 840 x 2 = 1,680

8-hour shifts per day840 x 3 = 2,520

For one 200-bed focused unit:

200 divided by 5 = 40 physicians x 14 focused units

= 560 physicians at

12-hour shifts per day 560 x 2 = 1,120

8-hour shifts per day 560 x 3 = 1,680

Total number of physicians required for 42 focused units

1,120 + 840 + 560 = 2,520 physicians at

12 hour shifts 2,520 x 2 shifts = 5,040

8-hour shifts 2,520 x 3 shifts = 7,560

Plus, part time at ¼ full time 12 hour 5,040 ÷ 4 = 1,260

8 hour 7,520 ÷ 4 = 1,880

The 1,260 12 hour or 1,880 8-hour part-time physicians would cover days off, sick days, continuous medical education time and vacations.

Total number of Focused Centres of Excellence physicians

8 hour shifts 7,060 + 1,880 = 8,940

12 hour shifts 5,040 + 1,260 = 6,300

Many more physicians will find work in other areas of health care in the IQSA system.

Summary

1. The number of patients to be cared for at all Focused Centres of Excellence = **1,134,000**

2. The total number of specialist physicians required for all Focused Centres of Excellence

8-hour shift: 8,940

12-hour shift: 6,300

3 The number of physician specialists required to alternate work between a focused specialist and a virtual consult specialist if the ratio is 1 VCS to five FS

8-hour shifts: 8,940 FS divided by 5 VCS = 1788

12-hour shifts: 6300 FS divided by 5 VCS = 1260

The above calculation would depend on the ratio of VCS to FS that was decided upon.

Please note: the number of physicians required for Focused Centres of Excellence and the H2C will be higher because of sick time and vacation variables. The H2C (health consultation centre) would require a ratio of one consultation specialist per five focused specialists at Focused Centres of Excellence. Some other physicians required and not factored in will be needed to provide services such as hematology, anesthesiology, radiology, pathology, research, and development. These are services that will continue to be needed in many categories of care at Focused Centres of Excellence as they may be an integral part of the treatment of many conditions.

All Focused Centres of Excellence have FS (focused specialists) that function as the admitting/attending focused specialist. The primary duty of the admitting/attending FS at a Focused Centre of Excellence is to care for five focused in-patients and video conference with five patients or their care provider or both, at one of the following locations: a tertiary care centre, a primary care centre, a primary emergency care centre, or a hospital emergency department. All video conferencing would be done through virtual consulting specialists at the H2C (health consultation centre). Consulting with specialists at the H2C takes place regarding diagnosis and treatment planning, daily charting, and assisting the admitting physician in overseeing residents and medical students. Any rapid change in the patient condition or planned treatment at a Focused Centre of Excellence would result in a consult.

There is a lot of work required to determine the category, size, location, and staffing levels of each type of Focused Centre of Excellence. Illness or injury occur in varying numbers resulting in the need for some focused units to be larger or smaller than others.

In the example above, care has been divided into three-unit sizes. This would allow for greater dispersion throughout the province and lessen any negative effect on local economies. This is a very important consideration as a hospital in any community is a major employer. Reforming health care to focus on specialized health care in only a few communities would cause unnecessary hardship and opposition to the plan. Health care jobs and the income generated are a substantial source of employment and income in many communities. These communities depend on employment that the health care sector provides to keep their economies running.

The gradual shift to more centralized care has been occurring for some time and has resulted in many smaller community hospitals losing funding and staffing as services were moved to larger centres. This sometimes occurred because of staffing requirements or the high cost of some equipment and the cost-utilization factor of such equipment. Sometimes equipment would become outdated before treating the number of patients required to see a reasonable return on the invested cost of the equipment. An example of this is a machine costing $100,000 and it is estimated that each patient treatment on the machine should cost $20. It would take 5,000 treatments to reach the $20 number. Fewer and the cost goes up per patient goes up. More patients treated and the cost goes down.

With the new IQSA system, health care will be distributed evenly throughout all IQSA RR in the province. This will result in maintaining the economic and health benefits currently provided by local health care, while encompassing benefits derived from a large coordinated province-wide system. This is possible because of technology and the internet's ability to connect people through live voice, video and imagery. The use of Focused

Centres of Excellence will mean health care will not be as diversified locally as it was before the change, but the current number of local beds within each hospital and the IQSA RR will be maintained.

These larger units will be needed to provide the very best care for patients in an efficient and efficacious manner but will also justify the huge expense of purchasing and possibly developing new technologies We must keep in mind that science is rapidly expanding our ability to treat illness and injury in new ways. Laparoscopic surgery is already replacing many other types of surgery and, with use of a robotic arm, its precision increases and it is less invasive. This type of surgery will give way to internet surgery meaning the patient and the surgeon can be miles apart. Such equipment is very costly and something only very large units could justify purchasing. This type of change is just the beginning. A new age is coming and the question will be: is the system ready, or will it fall further behind?

Health care that is "system ready" meaning 24/7/365 will correct many of the deficiencies in the current system. To engage the system ready approach will require large numbers of patients to employ the specialists around the clock. King-size focused units can do this. A drawback of this new system is that it will require the separation of patients from their families and loved ones for short periods of time as some treatment may require travel. This is sometimes the case today as well, but the future will see this happen with greater frequency. Depending on the situation, appropriate care may involve quite some travel distance, and then the patient may return to their local tertiary community hospital to convalesce if extended care is required. Making travel for care commonplace may be a trade-off in receiving faster, higher quality, lower-cost care. A trade-off, yes, but well worth it.

Deciding which IQSA RR will provide which categories (types) of care will be a collaborative decision-making process. Some categories of care may only have one unit in the province, but others may have more. As indicated in the prior example, if there are 42 in-patient focused units in the province, then each of the 14 IQSA RRs will have 3 focused units (one 200-bed, one 300-bed, and one 400-bed), with the option of up to 3 types of specialized care. The system is flexible, however, and it may be possible for a IQSA RR to specialize in only one category of care, dedicating all 900 of its beds to this. Such an option would depend on many factors such as need, staffing requirements, funding and bed availability.

The tertiary care centres will be community oriented, providing care, in most cases, to those that reside in the local area. Care at the tertiary hospital will be provided by nurses and other health care providers but no physicians will be located there. The FS physician that took care of the patient at the Focused Centre of Excellence will oversee care as a virtual FS, and will video conference with patients and staff at the tertiary care centre daily or more often as required.

All Focused Centres of Excellence provide a highly focused level of care. The VCS (virtual consult specialist) at the H2C located at each Focused Centre of Excellence will develop the specialized care plan template for standard care that outlines all care to be provided or a blank template for custom care that will need to be filled in with each step and used by the FS. The standard care plan is very specific outlining all steps to be taken and checked off as completed. The plan for custom care will be developed by the FS as soon as possible and may be developed while the patient is enroute to reduce the time required for treatment. Focused Centres of Excellence are short-term stay units covering one to four days before transfer out, if required, to a tertiary care hospital (formerly a community general hospital) or back to their residence. The current regional hospital in each IQSA RR will in most cases be the location of some or all Focused Centres of Excellence if it is large enough. Each IQSA RR in discussion with all other IQSA RRs, the hospital, and the ministry, will choose the categories of care (types) for their Focused Centres of Excellence.

For the purpose of this book, critical mass is defined as sufficient numbers of patients to employ specialists 24/7. Operating rooms will function around the clock, providing care to thousands of patients, not hundreds. In both medical and surgical units, close monitoring of patients will occur. All focused units may use AI to assist in accommodating this change.

Today's hospitals have small units (i.e., ICU) that do not have sufficient numbers of patients to consider "system ready" operation. Often there are no specialists onsite at night. These small units will be folded into the larger IQSA Focused Centres of Excellence. Those hospitals without focused units or beds in excess of focused unit needs will be designated as tertiary care community hospitals. In the past, much success occurred through the development of special units devoted to treating only one type of illness or injury. In Ontario, such examples include the sanatoriums that treated TB and polio, the Princess Margaret Cancer Centre, and the Shouldice Hernia Hospital. To establish a focused unit, care must be provided to enough patients to meet a threshold where many specialists can be kept busy 24/7.

The old idea of providing all care at the local level changed years ago. In the 1950s and 1960s, patients went to their community hospital for all care and most hospitals provided much the same range of care. Then in the 1970s and 1980s, care started to shift. The community hospital no longer provided all care but sent many patients to larger regional hospitals. Most small-town hospitals stopped delivering babies and doing surgery decades ago. This type of care was concentrated at the regional hospital level, with care provided by specialists. And now, the next step forward is to surpass regional care with a system designed to serve the province. This is accomplished with Focused Centres of Excellence, that are system ready. Large Focused Centres of Excellence have specialists onsite 24/7 to provide high intensity, complex, focused care for short periods of time and then the patient proceeds home, or if required, is transferred back to tertiary care nearest to their home.

No hospitals will close, and not much change externally should be required for regional or community hospitals to adapt to the requirements of a Focused Centre of Excellence. The units must be large enough to accommodate 24/7 care and to service the needs of the province. With the example provided above, no new beds will be required. The overall number of beds will remain the same. The current number of beds will be divided up into Focused Centre of Excellence beds and tertiary care beds.

The health care system needs to make a shift to 24/7 care with specialized focused units providing care according to illness or injury type. Not *location based*, as it is now, but *condition based*. The old style of treatment sometimes resulted in hospitals providing care that they did not routinely provide, and they often lacked the expertise to do so. They did this because there were no alternatives to the community hospital. People wrongly assumed their hospital could look after anything.

The change to Focused Centres of Excellence means that attending physicians will be very familiar with the condition and what needs to be done, and they will have provided that care copious times every year. This will be world class care for every patient no matter where they live in the province. Shifting all care to focused care will often mean that the patient will be required to travel some distance for care, but primary care, primary emergency care, tertiary care, along with emergency care, will still continue to be provided close to home, all guided virtually by focused specialists as required.

There is no substitute for experience. Experienced professionals provide better care and experience in a specialty is what the IQSA system is all about. Focused 24/7 units will provide medical students with the best resident experience where they can learn from specialists with abundant experience. And they will learn it in far less time than is normally required in today's system. In addition, with the province as a catchment, area physicians will have steady work. Few will have skills or knowledge atrophy due to periods of inactivity or when demand is low. Instead, practicing to the full extent of their training will benefit patients.

For focused excellence in care to occur, economies of scale must be achieved whether in medical care or surgical care. There must be sufficient numbers of patients requiring care in anyone category of care to engage physician specialists 24/7. If demand is not high enough, the objectives of Focused Centres of Excellence as laid out in this book will not be achieved and the system will not function at peak efficiency. This does not mean that a unit must be located only where demand is high. With a good transportation network, high volume units utilizing economies of scale can be located anywhere that staffing needs can be met. This may take time for staff to be trained. If a Focused Centre of Excellence is not quite meeting patient flow to reach the critical mass needed to enable economies of scale, a solution to this is presented in Chapter 12.

Today, intensive care units in general hospitals may be providing care to any number of different conditions. A system of Focused Centres of Excellence operating 24/7 will mean that each Focused Centre will have its own intensive care unit (ICU) for care in the designated specialty, with internists and other specialists as required. Most patients at the Focused Centre of Excellence would stay approximately four days or less, however those patients in the focused ICUs may have a longer stay.

Creating a system where all in-patient care is provided by Focused Centres of Excellence specialists that concentrate on the treatment of only one condition, is a major advance over the type of care we have now, which is largely unorganized with many types of care provided within many IQSA RRs while some types of care may not be provided there at all. Organizing care through the use of Focused Centres of Excellence geared to a province-wide approach (or larger), will change health care immensely, providing everyone with the best care available. The change will also lend itself to new processes that will streamline the work, introduce efficiencies, boost quality and efficacy, and increase speed and volume, all while lowering per patient treatment cost through faster treatment. Some of these advances will be managed in some Focused Centres of Excellence by creating sub specialities. An example might be where the focused trauma unit has a division for head trauma.

In the current system, the administration has worked very hard at trying to accommodate everyone as close to home as possible, no matter what their condition. But to continue this approach into the future is not economically feasible and does not always achieve the best results. Providing all care close to home requires more facilities, more staff, and more equipment to care for small numbers of patients. Essentially, much of the high-cost equipment does not operate around the clock. Having idle equipment and unused space costs time and money; it delays treatment and allows progression of disease and worsening of injuries. Having only parts of the system geared toward 24/7 service is how the system has operated for decades, and its problems have become clear. Change is needed and focused units will bring that change.

It is the large, Focused Centres of Excellence that will capitalize on the economy of scale. All aspects of our modern lives have shifted from the small mom-and-pop type businesses or facilities to the large giant-size centres. The small country grocery store with little variety has transformed into a superstore selling thousands of products and drawing customers from a very large catchment area. The local drug store has grown many times in size sometimes selling food products, medical products, cosmetics and increasingly sells its products online; and the garage mechanic has increased the number of bays and added a shop that sells much more than just tires. Even diagnosing car problems is shifting online and a computer program adjusts the engine. It has been postulated that if we did away with these new super-sized stores and electronics that have grown to meet the needs of today, the number of mom-and-pop stores required to replace them would be substantial and not practical. The needs of today can only be met through giant super stores and today they are called big box stores. This type of approach needs to be applied to health care also. So far it has not because we, as consumers of health care, believe that it must be provided locally. But this is not necessarily the case. The system can be structured to be both local *and* province wide.

What we have now is a collection of many small (mom-and-pop) health care units. They are small units with fixed operating hours and small staffing numbers that are unable to provide physician 24/7 service continuously or to care for large numbers of patients. Small units make up our current system that is not equipped to provide care when a patient requires it because the system concentrates on a specific local or regional geographic area. That area generally has small numbers of specific medical conditions or injuries The best professionals cannot be located in every town and no single health care provider is able to do it all or to be there at all times. In some areas of the province, it was best not to have your heart attack on the weekend or during summer break, or to have your car accident in a small town where the doctor was on call or where some paramedics were not as well trained as others. This is not to say that you would not receive care because in most cases, staff were on call for such occurrences. However, it does take time to assemble an "on-call team," which in some cases, only prepared the patient to transfer out to where another team was ready and assembled.

We have made progress on many inequities in the system but on some, we have not. They are ingrained in the *type of system* that we have, and the only solution is to change the system. Some may call this radical change, but I see it as more of a trend in care just as the small mom-and-pop stores gave way to larger and larger superstores. This same approach would be used in the IQSA system. That is, upgrading care by specializing and increasing focused unit size to take advantage of economies of scale. Introducing virtual consult specialists in the new online system might be compared to big-box stores opening virtual online stores. Both online stores and remote treatment by online physicians are relatively new services that are extending their reach 24/7. These steps are only part of the solution. Improving the processes within the reconfigured system will still need to take place.

Let's look at an example in Winnipeg. There, an orthopedic surgical unit works in a new way to a new standard that allows for faster quality care. The surgical unit employs a physician assistant to assist the orthopedic surgeon in the OR when they are doing hip replacements. The assistant prepares the patient, explaining the procedure, brings them into the OR, and begins the surgery with an incision to open the patient. At this point, the surgeon who has just finished in another OR, comes in and begins the work of replacing the hip. Once done, the physician assistant will then return to suture the incision closed while the surgeon is on their way to the next prepared patient. This allowed the surgeon to greatly increase the number of hip replacements. These highly efficient services provided by the physician assistant (and nurse anaesthetist) need to be more widely employed in the future.

Focused unit efficiency depends on high volumes. Surgeons today are not practicing their work at the volume required for future super efficiency. Many only get OR time once or twice a week and often all steps in the procedure are reserved for the surgeon when there may be some steps that could be done just as effectively by other professionals.

Chapter Highlights

The IQSA system will mean a shift to 24/7 Focused Centres of Excellence. A meeting of all IQSA RR authorities, the ministry, and hospitals will help decide what specialized services are provided and where. Each IQSA RR may chose a maximum of three specialties in which they will concentrate their efforts to excel. The focused units may be 200-, 300-, or 400-bed units but only a maximum of three units per IQSA RR. All other beds within the IQSA RR will be tertiary care beds.

The general hospitals of today have become very complex organizations. Managing all the different aspects and keeping on top of all the information has become very difficult. Dividing up the health care spectrum into specialized Focused Centres of Excellence units and increasing the size of the units will reduce the management complexity for each IQSA RR. They can then concentrate on being the best in fewer areas of care. The future lies in focused units for in-patients.

CHAPTER 5

IQSA Divisions of Care

Not all sectors of health care will change to the same degree. Nursing homes, birthing centres, diagnostic imaging clinics, physiotherapy clinics, cardio clinics, assessment teams, and others may all function much the same as they do now except that physician contact, if required, is with a virtual focused specialist at the Focused Centres of Excellence. Chapter 3 explained the Focused Centres of Excellence. This chapter explains other sectors that are greatly impacted by the change to the IQSA system.

In this plan nurse practitioners will gradually increase primary care provision, taking over the office care that family physicians provided. This will happen slowly as family physicians transition to a specialty. Nurse practitioners will work in nurse practitioner-led clinics (such as those in Sudbury), which employ a type of team approach where there may be a variety of health care providers such as dietitians, social workers, and registered nurses.

Nurse practitioners are not trained to do all that a family physician was trained to do, such as delivering babies. Nurse practitioner-led clinics are not new. What is new is that in the future, this will be the only way that primary care will be delivered. But this is not the big change. It is the way in which the care is delivered that will improve care for all patients.

Technology will play a much bigger role, linking each and every site when required (primary care site, primary emergency care site, emergency department, Focused Centres of Excellence, birthing centre, assessment team, tertiary hospitals, imaging centres, and others), to focused specialists 24/7 through consult specialists at the H2C.

Nurse practitioner clinics will be widely distributed throughout the province, however, there will be fewer than there are doctors' offices. This is because they are open 24/7 and will be staffed by more than one nurse practitioner thus, will be able to treat more patients than a single doctor in their office with typically limited hours. This will make these new clinics far more economical to operate. They will require far less real estate than all current family physicians' offices combined, that they will replace, and less real estate should have less associated costs including the following. Associated support staff (secretaries, cleaners, etc.), office supplies, and utility bills with more explained by Jeremy Petch, et al, (paraphrased) in a report showing a wide range of overhead cost with emergency physicians reporting the least at 12.5% to the highest being in ophthalmology at 42.5%. [xix]

Another advantage is that supplies for all these nurse practitioner clinics can be purchased in bulk with expected savings. All these measures taken together will add up to substantial savings. But this is not the best part of 24/7 service. Patients will benefit greatly from having access when they need the system and not when the system is ready to accept them. That's how it works now, except for emergency cases most of the time. With the new system, however, anytime anyone needs primary care they will know that a nurse practitioner's clinic will be open. They can receive care quickly by booking an appointment through Ontario Telehealth. In addition, nurse practitioner clinics are team staffed, meaning that patients can receive care from other allied health care providers without having to go elsewhere. All nurse practitioner clinics are tied into the system through the H2C. This is a vital link and will greatly benefit patients and the system.

The IQSA (integrated, quality, sustainable, accessible) system will build on change in primary care that has already started. Nurse practitioner-led primary care clinics already exist but now will be expanded throughout the province and be open 24/7. Longer hours of operation will result in fewer clinics needed and faster service. Patients will not have to wait. When they need the system, the system is ready for them. The IQSA system ensures that primary care is "system linked and ready" when the patient needs it. Strategically located, they will improve service while reducing costs.

The change to nurse practitioner-led clinics with a team approach has to do with the way they will be managed and how they fit precisely into the IQSA system, providing seamless, efficient, high-quality health care. Always linked into the system means nurse practitioners will have guaranteed access to specialists whenever consultation or admission is required. Time is always a factor with care and with the time to access specialists and the time required for admission greatly reduced, the result will be a higher probability of a speedier recovery

The nurse practitioner will not be working alone nor will anyone else in the system. Support for health care providers and thus their patients will be there 24/7. The IQSA system produces a methodical, organized process for the best in-patient care, increasing harmony and reducing stress. Contact with specialists is accomplished through the health consultation centre (H2C) and is the same protocol for all health care providers. The H2C is a facility that is staffed by virtual consultation specialists that monitor, record, and consult on all patient care between health care providers and the specialists at the Focused Centres of Excellence. The consistent protocol for contact will reduce stress for health care providers and improve care for patients.

As the shift from family physicians' changes over to other primary care providers, facilities may need to be built. In some cases, facilities that were publicly funded for use by physicians could be used by nurse practitioners and others, but in some cases an investment may be required. Just as physician offices were numerous, primary care facilities will be numerous but not as abundant as doctors' offices because of their 24/7 operation and team approach.

All emergency departments will remain in operation as they are now and they will be staffed by emergency physicians and other staff as required. The rest of the hospital now becomes a tertiary care hospital minus the space required for those hospitals with Focused Centres of Excellence. Emergency departments would continue to be managed by the hospital board. The new IQSA system divides up emergency care into care that requires admission and primary emergency care that does not. The emergency department at the hospital, staffed by emergency physicians, cares for those types of patients requiring admission. Managing the emergency department in this way will make a notable difference. Emergency departments will be able to manage the flow of patients with much greater efficiency, producing greater satisfaction among patients and health care providers. Those that do not need emergency admission would be treated by paramedics at primary emergency care centres. Both are open 24/7. In the current system, the only facility open 24/7 is the emergency department. If we provided care 24/7 at other facilities, wait times would drop and overcapacity in the emergency department would be reduced.

Deciding where to go might cause some public confusion in the beginning, but this could be lessened if all patients needing emergency care or primary emergency care are required to call Telehealth Ontario to receive an ID number. Telehealth Ontario is a nurse staffed and operated phone line already in existences. They will assess your health problems and direct you to the appropriate health care provider. Having all patients contact Telehealth has additional benefits, especially in a crisis. If one primary emergency care centre, emergency department or other facility is at capacity, patients could be diverted to other facilities operating under capacity. Any information given to Telehealth will be forwarded via the VCS to the appropriate facility.

The emergency department emergency physician may contact the H2C at any time to request admission of a patient but it is still up to the FS to decide on treatment and if admission is required. Nurse practitioners at primary care sites or paramedics at primary emergency care sites may also contact the H2C at anytime, but are mandated to do so when the patient has been treated twice without improvement and is on the third visit for the same condition. In this type of situation, a consult is mandatory unless it is considered an emergency. Once contacted, the focused specialist may prescribe or change medication or prescribe another form of treatment or recommend elective admission or emergency admission. Emergency transfers will be done by the local ambulance service, land or air as is currently done. If an obvious emergency case arrives at any site, an ambulance is immediately requested and the patient is sent to the emergency department. The VCS is then contacted as soon as possible.

Paramedics will gradually ramp up to provide all primary emergency care service, with patients being diverted from hospital emergency departments as primary emergency centres are established. A few procedures or treatments will require additional training and in future, a university degree program for paramedics will be advantageous for primary emergency care paramedics. Afterward, a new designation may have them named paramedic practitioners. Paramedics are specialized in the treatment of patients in emergency situations "in the field." However, their expertise is beginning to be utilized with "out-of-hospital" care since the introduction of community paramedics.

Paramedics are not trained in all that a family physician or an emergency physician can do. Rather, they are trained in only a portion of that, and this is why they are specialists. It is interesting to note that paramedics were one of the first groups of health care providers to be in constant contact with virtual physicians through the ambulance on-board communication system. This will help make them more at ease working in the IQSA system.

One of the reasons why the ambulance communication system originated was because of the need for emergency departments to receive information on what was coming in. This allowed the department necessary preparation time as patients were enroute. The primary care clinics bring out the best in nurse practitioners, and primary emergency care centres will bring out the best in paramedics. Primary emergency care centres will differ from urgent care centres by the fact that they are staffed by paramedics and are open 24/7. Primary emergency care facilities would need to be established. The location of the primary emergency care centres would, whenever possible, correspond to the same location where there is an ambulance base and a nurse practitioner clinic if possible.

Although it should not happen, a situation may arise when a patient arrives at a primary emergency centre that may require emergency care. Emergency patients will be transferred by ambulance to the closest emergency department immediately, to be stabilized. In this case, the VCS may be contacted when the patient is enroute to the emergency department. The primary emergency care paramedic will contact the VCS at H2C. A video conference between the paramedic, the emergency physician, and a focused specialist will be set up. The consult specialist will monitor, record, and consult on every case providing every patient with a second opinion. As always, the consult specialist waits until the end of the video conference when the FS will ask the VCS if there are any questions, comments, or concerns. If there are no concerns, the consulting specialist only needs to say that they concur. If advice is provided, it will be based on standard evidence-based care but will not be binding on the emergency physician or the FS.

Both emergency department care and primary emergency care, along with primary care, are in frequent contact with focused specialists at the Focused Centres of Excellence through the H2C. All may contact a VCS at the H2C and request a focused specialist video conference at any time.

The primary emergency care centres may also use a team approach similar to current nurse practitioner clinics. This is when other health care provides may be located at the site creating a team. Different types of teams with different professionals will provide options that may differ from location to location. Work at finding the right combinations for the locality will need to be done. Both paramedics and nurse practitioners are specialists with their own fields of expertise. Nurse practitioners provide clinic/team-based primary care and paramedics provide clinic/team-based primary emergency care. All primary care and primary emergency care centres will be open 24/7. These two groups will need to be able to consult with and refer to specialists as required without encountering problems that exist today, such as the overbooked specialists unable to take a referral for months.

How do we correct for this problem? Increasing the number of specialists with this plan will enable a consult within minutes and the wait for actual treatment at a Focused Centre of Excellence should lessen from months to days for elective cases. Coordinating the new system of specialists and the care they provide would be done through a new service referred to as the virtual consult specialist (VCS) which makes up the Health Consultation Centre (H2C). More about this in the next chapter.

The IQSA system provides the best care, by the right health care provider, in the right place around the clock. All admitted patients will receive care at Focused Centres of Excellence and some may have extended care provided at tertiary care hospitals where nursing care is emphasized. Physicians will not be at the tertiary care hospitals. Patients at tertiary care hospitals will be cared for virtually by the same focused specialists that looked after them at the Focused Centres of Excellence.

The role that community hospitals play is recognized as an important part of the foundation of many communities and contributes greatly to the healing process. That is why they remain a vital part of the IQSA system. But they do so with a new mandate and transition to become tertiary care hospitals.

They provide the type of care that some patients need in the familiar setting of their own community. No type of diagnosis or design of a treatment plan is done at a tertiary care hospital. Those functions are performed at the Focused Centres of Excellence by focused specialists. What this means is that to be admitted to a tertiary care hospital the patient must have been treated at a Focused Centre of Excellence first. Nurses at the tertiary hospital would be consulting with a focused specialists daily or more often regarding patients that were sent to them by the focused specialist. The tertiary care hospital would be for those that live in the vicinity. The tertiary care hospital in this aspect would be reminiscent in a small way of the cottage hospitals that were present in England in the late 1800s and early 1900s. They were small, built for the local population but today would be providing excellent nursing care video linked province wide. That is the idea behind tertiary care hospitals.

In 2012 there were approximately 31,000 hospital beds in Ontario. Twenty-three categories (types) of care for Focused Centres of Excellence have been identified in a previous chapter. In that example, 42 Focused Centres of Excellence provide the care required. That leaves 18,400 beds for tertiary care hospitals. That is over half the beds at that time, in the system that would be dedicated to tertiary care. This is defined as care for those patients requiring additional care beyond the maximum four days at a Focused Centres of Excellence. These beds would continue to be located in all the hospitals that do not have Focused Centres of Excellence and may include some that do if the focused units do not require all the beds. All care in tertiary care hospitals would be provided by the same types of health care providers currently, except for physicians. The physicians looking after these patients would be the same focused specialists that took care of those patients at the Focused Centres of Excellence, and they would continue to do so by video conferencing.

The video conferencing between the focused specialist and patient, or between the focused specialist and another health care provider, would be somewhat similar to the current system provided at Health Sciences North in Sudbury. The program there is called the virtual critical care program. In that program, physicians in rural or remote areas of the northeast use video conferencing to consult on treatment with a specialist in Sudbury. The program allows the specialist to see and talk to the patient to determine the best course of treatment or to discuss cases with the attending physician or follow up with prescribed care. The main difference between this program and the program at the tertiary care hospital being proposed is that the specialist would be video conferencing with other types of health care providers, primarily nurses, not physicians.

At this point, the design of the IQSA health care system covers the same number of patients that can be treated in the old system and possibly a few more. This means that the number of beds need not change so hospitals will not have the additional capital expenditure of adding new beds. The change is in how the beds are used. And that change is aimed toward specialization. Those hospitals that did provide a wide range of treatment will no longer do so.

The goal is to have integrated, quality, sustainable, and accessible care with each IQSA RR providing care at no more than three Focused Centres of Excellence, and no more than three categories of care. The IQSA system will be fully operational on a 24/7 basis providing care at a much faster pace than in the old system. The patient will begin receiving treatment much sooner. This means, for example, that if the patient began receiving treatment within 24 hours after admission in the past, it may now only take 8 hours or less depending on the time required for the patient to rest.

In our current system, each IQSA RR has smaller community hospitals providing care to the local population, but usually only one large regional hospital that provides services that the smaller community hospitals are unable to provide. This pattern of extending care to patients from smaller community hospitals to a larger regional hospital will now transition and extend care for patients from outside the IQSA RR. It will be accomplished through the Focused Centres of Excellence located in each IQSA RR where patients from anywhere in the province will receive highly complex, specialized, focused care. This method of care is not new. In fact, some hospitals in Ontario currently receive patients from the far reaches of the province for specialized care such as trauma. The Focused Centres of Excellence will usually be located at what was previously the regional hospital but maybe, wherever there are beds in sufficient number within the IQSA RR.

The future will be similar to today but it will also have distinct differences. The future of definitive health care will be specialists working to their highest and best function. This means that they must be employed at specialized units 24/7 and extend their reach to tertiary care hospitals through video conferencing. In this way, it could be said that the tertiary care hospitals are specializing also, being primarily a nursing hospital. The FS would now provide care virtually to their patients that they cared for at a Focused Centre of Excellence. As always this is done in conjunction with and through a VCS. The tertiary care hospitals would have a mix of patients needing many different types of care according to their condition. All patients requiring extended care would be cared for by the same FS and VCS that looked after them at the Focused Centre of Excellence. All hands-on care at the tertiary hospital is provided by nurses skilled in video conferencing with virtual FS's located at Focused Centres of Excellence.

Advancing the health care system so patients are able to receive the care they need when they need it means around the clock service. Not just a portion of the care but all of the care. A future with 24/7 service means large units caring for thousands of patients yearly, utilizing all the resources that have been brought together and never letting them sit idle. It does not make sense to have a 24/7 emergency department when other necessary components are not 24/7. It would be like having planes fly 24/7 but at the same time, have limited operating hours at airports. Or a restaurant open 24/7 but the kitchen closed at night.

Currently, each IQSA RR has several hospitals within its boundaries. As stated, all those hospitals without focused units will become tertiary care hospitals staffed only by nurses and other non-physician care providers. If the current hospitals within a IQSA RR are not large enough to accommodate the size of the Focused Centre of Excellence, then consideration will need to be given to expanding the site of the Focused Centre of Excellence. Those hospitals with Focused Centres of Excellence units may also have tertiary care hospital beds if space permits, but separate accounting books would be kept for each. The tertiary care hospitals and the Focused Centres of Excellence are managed by the current hospital board. The tertiary care hospital will follow the care plan that was developed at the Focused Centre of Excellence by the focused specialist. The care plan (chart) will have daily entries from the focused physician and tertiary staff that provide care to the patient. Any proposed changes to the plan will require a consult with the VCS before proceeding.

The future will be bright for the smaller tertiary hospitals. They will provide improved care for patients through virtual focused specialists. They will be more resourceful and integrated with the community (inviting private business to join the site). They have always been a hub of activity in the community and will become even more so. Over time they will develop their potential at partnering with the private sector to offset costs. This could be done by becoming a landlord for other community services related to health. As has been done at some hospital sites already. Some could invite a drug store to the site or a gym, other possibilities include a food court or gift shops or clothing stores for special needs. The list could be long. Income from the landlord-tenant relationship could be used to offset health care costs at the tertiary care hospital. None of this is new. Hospitals have had gift shops for decades and this has expanded over time at many sites making them an even greater hub of activity in the community. Even Tim Hortons can be found there sometimes.

Many other health care providers will continue to provide services at current facilities, including midwives at birthing centres, physiotherapists at clinics, X-ray and ultrasound technicians at medical imaging and independent laboratory sites, and nurses and personal support workers providing home care services etc. These sites will maintain communications with the patient's primary health care provider (the nurse practitioner). As an example, midwives will continue to look after uncomplicated maternity cases and most mothers will deliver at birthing centres. Midwives and their patients may also at times be in contact with obstetrician specialists at a Focused Centre of Excellence, and difficult cases or those anticipating problems will be transferred. All communication is through the H2C.

Chapter Highlights

A new approach to health care extends to the emergency department where emergency care is divided into emergency care for those patients that require admission, and primary emergency care provided by paramedics at primary emergency care centres for all those urgent cases that do not require admission.

Primary care will be provided by non-physician health care providers, primarily nurse practitioners working in teams with other health care providers. The teams are composed of those best suited to the needs of the community. Primary emergency care centres like all other sectors of the IQSA system are open 24/7 and are staffed by paramedics and other team members possibly virtually, based on community needs. Emergency departments will continue as they are.

CHAPTER 6

Coordination of the System

The IQSA Health Care System will be composed of all specialists. The next step will be to determine how the specialists and the system will function. There are two divisions in IQSA that coordinate the system. They are the health consultation centre (H2C) and the health transport centre (HTC). Both will do coordination, with the former consulting and coordinating patient care between providers and the latter, coordinating the movement of patients between health care sites. Together along with all the specialists are at the heart of the best system possible, the IQSA health care system.

The health consultation centre is composed of many virtual consult specialists (VCS) from many different specialties. A small H2C will be located at the same site as every Focused Centre of Excellence Focused Specialists will rotate work between working as a focused specialist and as a virtual consult specialist. A small group of VCSs will form the virtual diagnostic team (VDT) that can assist with difficult diagnosis. This will make it a multi-site service but it operates as though there is only one site.

The VCS will monitor, record, and consult on the diagnosis, treatment, and care of patients, providing a second opinion, but they do not make the final treatment decision. All sites are linked together as one to provide the type of specialist required. They oversee the creation, access, and storage of patient electronic medical records (EMR). They assist with development of care pathways, medical directives for evidence-based standard care, and create benchmarks. They assure *standard care* is the best evidence-based care, that it is updated as required, and that *custom care* is as safe and as efficacious as possible, and that all care for a patient is coordinated between health care providers at different units and other sectors of the health care system. In addition to the duties outlined above, the VCS oversees the IT (information technology) system that tracks such things as patient cost per day and cost per procedure, including quality performance indicators. Statistics generated will enable reports on quality assurance among other statistics. It will also provide regular feedback on performance to health care providers, including physicians, to enable them to improve care. The IT system does more than provide real-time electronic medical records. It also provides documentation templates, reminders, and alerts, especially for drug interactions. And of course, because the IT system is provided through the VCS, it also may assist with clinical-decision support.

The following are the steps taken in a typical patient-care algorithm call to a focused specialist

1. When a call comes in to the H2C, the caller identifies themselves and will request a consultation with a specific type of specialist. It will be up to the first VCS to confirm the type of specialist required. They will do this by video conferencing with the primary care provider and reviewing the patient chart that they have sent to the VCS.

2. After confirmation the VCS will check a roster to confirm the availability of the next three focused specialists of the type requested. Another roster will indicate the availability of a VCS of the same type as the focused specialist.

3. The new VCS will send a list of three focused specialists (FS) to the patient so they can choose one.

4. After receiving notice of the one chosen, a new VCS with the same credentials as the FS contacts the FS and sends them the patient's chart containing patient history, current chief complaint, current vital signs, medication list, any current tests completed, and any past EMR (electronic medical records) on file. Both the VCS and the FS will review the chart.

5. After the focused specialist has a short time to review the chart (10 to 15 minutes), they contact the VCS who then creates a video conference between the focused specialist, the patient, and the primary care provider. The patient will be told by the primary care provider that a second opinion on their condition will be given by another specialist. All video conferences and communications between providers or between providers and the VCS are monitored and video recorded by the VCS. During the video conference, the FS may virtually examine the patient while the health care provider assists with the "hands on."

6. At the end of the video conference, if the patient is to return home, the focused specialist will tell the patient what he may be able to do for the patient or talk about the next step they would like to take. If the patient is told to return home, a prescription may be given for medication, or additional tests may be requested, or some other type of treatment such as physiotherapy may be prescribed.

7. If the patient is told admission is required, the focused specialist will indicate to the patient whether it will be standard treatment or custom treatment. The focused specialist will privately confer with the VCS at the end of every video conference and

ask if there are any questions, comments, or concerns. This is done as a private conversation between the FS, VCS and the primary care provider. The VCS may reply with only one word, "Concur," meaning everything regarding proposed treatment is within standard care practice guidelines and is evidence based, or they may have any number of questions, or may advise further testing. The VCS does not speak to the patient, only to the FS, but is always in the background being as unobtrusive and as discreet as possible. Any advice given by the VCS is standard evidence-based care only.

8. The focused specialist will direct questions that the VCS may have to the patient or the primary care provider. Both the FS and VCS will take any answers into consideration. If a more intensive assessment of the patient is required, the focused specialist or the consult specialist may recommend more testing or may recommend the patient be seen by an assessment team. This will be arranged by the VCS.

9. If admission has been decided upon, the VCS will arrange for a bed at the focused specialist's Focused Centre of Excellence. They will also pass on a request for transport to the Health Transport Centre that will arrange transportation, if required, in which case the call would be transferred to a Health Transport Coordinator (HTC) for the primary care provider, or the primary emergency care provider, to speak with the HTC.

10. If the FS has chosen admission with a custom treatment plan, the focused specialist will submit an electronic copy outlining all steps in the proposed treatment. This may take some time and will be completed while the patient is enroute to the Focused Centre of Excellence. All custom treatment plans will be reviewed by the VCS who may make recommendations to

make the custom treatment as safe and efficacious as possible. If a standard treatment is decided on, the standard treatment template will be sent to the focused specialist. Each step in the treatment plan is already outlined. All that is required are signatures or password codes as the treatment outlined is completed. All recommendations made by the VCS whether for standard or custom treatment will not be mandatory, but all recommendations are recorded.

At times, VCSs act as patient care co-pilots, advising the care providers of the best course of action for evidence-based standard care and will critique custom care. This is to help assure the patient receives the best care that can be provided by the care providers, including paramedics, nurse practitioners, registered nurses, focused specialists, and others at any time of the day or night. At other times, they will act as patient care navigators, directing the patient from the primary care site to the proper location and the proper specialist for the care required 24/7. It is all part of maintaining quality. Additional tasks could be developed in the future. The VCS will not decide patient care and will not provide it, but will give a second opinion, highlighting specific care options where applicable. Any advice or information provided is not mandatory.

Fig. B

Condensed Patient Flowchart

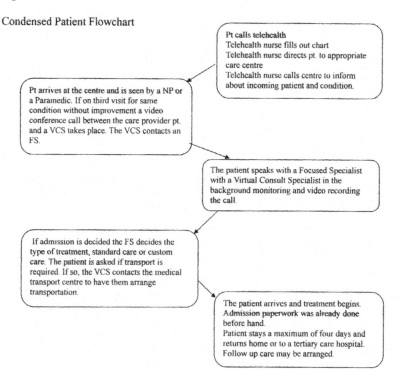

Pt calls telehealth
Telehealth nurse fills out chart
Telehealth nurse directs pt. to appropriate care centre
Telehealth nurse calls centre to inform about incoming patient and condition.

Pt arrives at the centre and is seen by a NP or a Paramedic. If on third visit for same condition without improvement a video conference call between the care provider pt. and a VCS takes place. The VCS contacts an FS.

The patient speaks with a Focused Specialist with a Virtual Consult Specialist in the background monitoring and video recording the call.

If admission is decided the FS decides the type of treatment, standard care or custom care. The patient is asked if transport is required. If so, the VCS contacts the medical transport centre to have them arrange transportation.

The patient arrives and treatment begins. Admission paperwork was already done before hand.
Patient stays a maximum of four days and returns home or to a tertiary care hospital. Follow up care may be arranged.

The VCS is virtual because they provide all consulting virtually over the internet. One responsibility of the virtual consult specialist is to assure that care between health care providers and health care sites transitions seamlessly. The consult specialist and the focused specialist (admitting/ attending specialist) have the same qualifications. They may both be at the same Focused Centre of Excellence or may be located at different sites. The focused specialist that was chosen will, in most cases be the only phy-sician to attend to the patient during their stay at the Focused Centre of Excellence. Occasionally, some categories of care will have sub-specialists that may provide care. The consult specialist connects together primary care, primary emergency care, emergency care, focused care, and ter-tiary care.

The patient must give consent to the treatment plan whether standard or custom care. If they do not, they will be given one other option. A new appointment will be set up with the primary care provider and they will go through the same process again. The result may not be any different. It will depend on the decision of the new focused specialist.

The province has been divided up into areas referred to as IQSA Referral Regions. These areas correspond to the old Local Health Integration Networks that was disbanded. Some of these IQSA RRs already have an assessment team that assesses the patient to determine eligibility for hip or knee replacements. With the IQSA system, the assessment team may evaluate the patient virtually or in-person during their rounds. Rounds consist of the team travelling within the IQSA RR, visiting predetermined sites once a week or as required. Many IQSA RR areas will organize an assessment team if it will be of advantage. The team may consist of kinesiologists, physiotherapists, and others specially trained in specific assessments to meet the need. The team will then report back to the focused specialist through video conferencing arranged by the consult specialist or may enter written findings on the electronic medical record (EMR) requested through a VCS. A notification of this will be automatically sent to the consult specialist and the focused specialist.

Both specialists will check the patient's chart daily, the focused specialist to make or read progress notes entered by other health care providers, or to make changes or additions to the treatment plan, and the consult specialist to review entries to assure standard care is the best evidence-based care updated as required, and that custom care is as safe and efficacious as possible. Any changes to the treatment plan made by the focused specialist will always be in consultation with the consult specialist. All video conferencing connections, are made through the virtual consult specialist and are monitored and recorded. At the end of every video conference with the patient, the VCS will be asked by the focused specialist if there are any questions, comments, or concerns.

The consult specialist oversees the provision of two types of care. Standard care and custom care. Standard care is evidence-based care and is provided through a care plan that is laid out in a standard format with the care pathways (protocols), including the medical directives to be initialed or signed with a password code as completed by the focused specialist each step along the way. The chart will also require the initials or code of anyone else providing care. The code would be the same as a signature.

The consult specialist reviews the chart of each patient they have consulted on, at least once a day, while the patient proceeds through the system. This may be required more often if a change to the treatment plan is going to be made, in which case the focused specialist will contact the consult specialist before making the change. The consult specialist reviews each step and the result daily, or more frequently as required, to assure that standard care is the best evidence-based care, that it is updated as required, and the custom care is as safe and efficacious as possible. If the standard care plan is deviated from, the VCS will bring this to the attention of the FS and if it is not corrected, the VCS may designate the care as having changed to custom care and the FS will need to write up a treatment plan in detail.

The same consulting specialist and the same focused specialist (admitting/attending specialist) will oversee the care of the patient through their journey from primary care, to focused care, to tertiary care if required. Over time all specialists will have a better understanding of the standard evidence-based treatment protocols and will be able to decide quickly whether they will follow the standard treatment plan or decide on a custom treatment plan. A custom treatment plan is designed by the focused specialist and will be reviewed by the VCS with the understanding that this may be a new type of treatment. All care plans will guide the care that the patient receives not unlike a flight plan used in the airline industry. The plan can be changed by the focused specialist, but reasons for the change, including possible advantages and drawbacks, need to be explained to the virtual consult specialist (VCS) after which the VCS can provide a non-binding opinion. Large changes may require a switch from standard care to custom care. This is a departure from the current system. There is no care plan written in advance, although the physician would have a mental image of where they are going based on their treatment and findings. This approach can work but opens the door to possible omissions and errors.

Many errors that occur in health care are process errors (defined as any deviation or omission in the process that may or may not cause harm) that can be greatly reduced through the IQSA Health Care System. All standard care evidence-based pathways and medical directives will be written down in advance to allow for all to see what has been done and what needs to be completed. All contact between health care providers goes through a VCS that assigns one VCS to each patient. The same consult specialist and focused specialist follows the patient through the system whenever possible. All patient care among different providers is coordinated and all information is available as required and requested. The VCS maintains oversite of EMRs and all patient-care charting including standard and custom care. All contact between health care providers is monitored and recorded with the consult specialist providing a non-binding second opinion at the end of every video conference. The second opinion provided by the consult specialist may result in only one word – "concur"– or may result in many varied recommendations. But it will always be evidence based and non-binding. Any standard care deviation on a scale from 1 to 10, will be noted with 1 being a minor deviation and 10 a major deviation.

An emergency admission video conference may originate from any place in the system where the patient is located. The video conference may be between the emergency physician and the primary care provider

(Nurse Practitioner, Paramedic) if the patient is at a primary care site; or may be between an emergency physician and the focused specialist if, after treatment at the emergency department, the patient requires admission. A video call may also originate at a tertiary care hospital when a registered nurse requires a consult with an FS. All emergency admissions are transferred by ambulance, be it land or air as is done now.

When compared to the airline industry, some of the consult specialist duties might at times be considered navigator duties and at other times, co-pilot duties. As a navigator, the consult specialist would assist the patient as they receive care from multiple care givers at multiple sites: from a nurse practitioner at a primary care site, to an emergency room physician, to a focused specialist at a Focused Centre of Excellence, to a nurse that specializes in virtual collaboration at a tertiary care hospital. For the primary care provider and the focused specialists (admitting/attending specialist), the consult specialist would act as co-pilot to assure that the care plans are followed and the treatment provides the greatest benefit. Additional duties for the consult specialist may include checking for drug interactions or doing as Queens Hospital in New York did. There they monitor antibiotic use to curtail overuse and consult with physicians to see if alternatives might be used. As a result, they found that the number of antibiotic-resistant bacterium has dropped among their patients.

Another advantage to having more specialists means that specialists can rotate work between the Focused Centres of Excellence and the health consultation centre (H2C). The H2C will be pivotal in the overall function of the IQSA Health Care System and will bring exciting innovation. The H2C will provide service to the whole province.

The IQSA system will depend on electronic medical records (EMR). All patient information will be stored on electronic medical records (EMR). All video recording will be added to the EMR but can only be accessed through a separate password provided by the VCS if needed. This information will be accessible to health care providers while providing care to the patient, but it must be requested through H2C. Those jurisdictions that have developed EMRs have found the process a difficult, expensive endeavour. So, by extending the advantage to include more patients from other locations, maybe outside of the province, the taxpayer would benefit through the time and money saved in the development and implementation of creating a new EMR.

All patients will receive a barcode or QR code to track their movement and care. Codes have also proven effective in assuring that patients receive the correct medication. The new EMR system in conjunction with a central bed registry, both managed by the H2C, will improve efficiency. The registry will list all Focused Centre of Excellence beds, including ICU beds and tertiary hospital beds.

Creating a truly 21st century system means applying advantages that some businesses now employ. Larger businesses can serve greater numbers of customers and are generally able to do it at a lower cost. Purchasing in bulk and automating services, when possible, reduce costs, but one study reported by Jacqueline LaPointe indicates saving through economy of scale in a range of 15 to 30 percent but some do not see the saving and are left with additional costs.[xx] IQSA is taking a system that is already large and connecting it in a way to realize savings. The system has to be designed for saving or it won't happen.

There must be a means of linking together all health care in the province. To combine the advantage of large business (Focused Centres of Excellence), with the advantage of small business (tertiary care hospitals), to in fact make it one system. In the United States, hospital corporations are becoming larger mostly through mergers and acquisitions.

Many hospitals already specialize in specific procedures and treatments but provide these services to a small number of patients. None work at an integrated system to the degree that the IQSA system does. Ontario has a tremendous advantage already with province-wide insurance that covers the entire population. If we take advantage of that and create units that specialize province wide, but make them much larger and expand their catchment area to the whole province the system would be able to enlist the patient numbers required to make the system work efficiently, effectively, and efficaciously for both the patient, the taxpayer, and the health care provider.

Tertiary care hospitals will serve the local population only and will be managed by the same board that currently manages the local hospital. Each hospital board will remain and will also manage the large Focused Centres of Excellence located at their site. The H2C and HTC will link the IQSA system together and be funded directly by the province. The rest of the system will be funded indirectly by the province through the IQSA RR and their local hospital boards. The IQSA RR is composed of all hospital CEOs in the region that would meet once a year or as required. To be admitted to a tertiary care hospital the patient must have first been treated at a Focused Centre of Excellence. Work at the tertiary care hospital does not provide a diagnosis and does not design a treatment plan. These tasks are done at the Focused Centres of Excellence. The tertiary care hospital will provide care during recovery for all that require it. A bed registry for all beds in Ontario will be kept at the H2C for use by the VCS. It will provide information on bed location, bed type (focused care beds, intensive care beds, or tertiary care beds), and bed occupancy. When a focused specialist requires additional recovery care for their patient after treatment at the Focused Centre of Excellence, the H2C will arrange for a bed at a tertiary care site.

There are four ways that a patient may start their health care journey. The most common method would be through a primary care clinic staffed by nurse practitioners and possibly other care providers. The other methods include a primary emergency care centre staffed by paramedics and possibly other care providers; a hospital emergency department staffed by emergency physicians and other care providers. And the fourth method, much less common, will be through a primary care family physician/specialist. All providers may contact H2C voluntarily at any time for consultation but some are mandated to do so during the third visit for the same problem when treatment has not resulted in an improvement.

If a patient is an emergency case and is not at a hospital emergency department, the patient would be transferred there immediately. The primary care provider (nurse practitioner, paramedic, primary care family/specialist physician) would contact H2C and pass on all information at the first opportunity. The H2C would then pass this on to the emergency department. Once the patient is stabilized at the emergency department, H2C is contacted, and admission may be arranged. If the patient is still classified as an emergency, an ambulance would transfer the patient by either land or air.

Change in the health care system is needed for many reasons and one among them is the amount of information in the medical field that has to be managed by health care professionals. This information has exploded and shows no sign of slowing down. Increasing the number of specialists in the manner described, and by creating a virtual consulting team of health care specialists, will enable health care providers to keep pace with the massive amounts of new information. There may also be more sub-specialists to assist in this work, increasing the possibility of new, more effective treatment under consideration.

With this plan, there will be enough specialists to create a fundamentally new type of service. Known as the virtual consult specialist (VCS) or consult specialist (CS) for shortform. It consists of a large group of specialists that will provide a second opinion through virtual consulting. They will never come into actual contact with the patient. The ratio of VCS specialists to focused specialists (admitting specialists) will need to be worked out, but a ratio of approximately one virtual consulting specialist (VCS) for every five focused specialists may work. The IQSA system has consulting specialists alternating between working as VCSs and working as focused specialists at a Focused Centre of Excellence.

Training family physicians to become specialists will increase the number of specialists and allow for some to work providing consultation. Others may work as family physicians/specialists after they become specialists, if there is not a position open for them immediately. Some may continue with this arrangement because they like the variety of work. Their names will be placed on a waiting list for full-time specialist employment. Accommodation by allowing some specialists to work at being both a specialist and a family physician may only be considered if the Focused Centres of Excellence do not run short of full-time specialists.

Having a virtual consult physician has proven very effective in the Ontario air ambulance system where they are employed. They provide a seamless and integrated system that improves the health care experience for the patient. The physicians that have this duty are referred to colloquially as "doc in a box." The consultation takes place between the "doc in a box" and physicians at sending facilities, receiving facilities, and paramedics on a regular basis while patients are being transferred between health care facilities by paramedics with the Ontario air ambulance system.

This was started because the Ontario air ambulance service (known as Ornge) had a problem. It was taking too long to complete transfers. When the helicopter landed at the hospital to pick up a patient, the paperwork was not always complete, the patient was not always prepared properly for air transport, patient care was not consistent between the sending hospital, the air ambulance, and the receiving hospital, and on arrival, the patient was sometimes required to spend long periods of time in the emergency department of the receiving hospital before being moved to the unit where they were booked.

These problems were cleared up when the "docs in a box" was hired and dedicated to the air ambulance system. The Ornge website explains that transport medicine physicians (docs in a box) collaborate with physicians to meet organizational objectives. They do this at an air ambulance communication centre where they maintain radio contact with air ambulances and use phones and computers to coordinate care between the sending facility, the receiving facility, and the paramedics.

A request for an air ambulance transfer would come into the central ambulance communication centre (CACC) and is then referred to Ornge where a transport medicine physician would then start medical treatment coordination. The sending facility would understand how to prepare the patient for flight and how to prepare the patient for direct admission without having to spend time in the emergency department of the receiving facility. The oversight has proven to be very effective in providing seamless top-notch care for the patient and less stress for all, plus quicker service. Applying this type of coordination of service to care throughout the province may bring about revolutionary improvements.

A new diagnostic team consisting of a few specialists would make up the virtual diagnostic team (VDT). The team would be part of the H2C. A few VCSs would comprise the internet-based team responding to calls for consultation on diagnosis of difficult cases from anywhere in the province. If required, a primary care provider would call a VCS and request the VCT for a diagnosis of their patient's problem. This may happen more so with a request coming from a focused specialist.

The provincial emergency ambulance, land and air system remains unchanged but is reserved for emergencies. Private patient transfer services, where they exist, may be called upon to do non-urgent transfers to the local transfer station (transport terminal) to rendezvous with the inter-city or inter-IQSA RR medical transport bus. Where private transfer services do not exist, local ambulance service may be called upon as they are now only now much less time will be required for the transfer because of the proximity to the transport terminal

The primary function of the virtual consult specialist (VCS) is to provide consultation with every primary health care provider and specialist that the patient would come into contact with, provide backroom services to navigate the patient through the health care system, and coordinate the system to improve flow. The VCS at the H2C would provide a second opinion for all patients. All charting is done by requesting the chart through the H2C. By this I mean that all health care providers would need to request access to the patient's electronic medical record (EMR) by requesting it from the consulting specialist. The ratio of consult specialists to focused specialists will need to be decided upon, but may be in the range of one consult specialist to every five focused specialists.

The VCS at the health consultation centre (H2C) will connect a primary health care provider to a focused specialist at a Focused Centre of Excellence site and will provide a second opinion on the patient's planned treatment. The primary provider might be a registered nurse practitioner, paramedic, emergency physician or family physician/specialist in transition, requesting consultation with the focused specialist. In the IQSA system, the focused specialist (admitting/attending physician) will do most of the attending unless there is a sub-specialist at the Focused Centre of Excellence who may be called upon. Referral to home care will be through the primary care provider but may be a suggestion from an FS.

The consult specialist would act as co-pilot providing an additional level of safety. They assure checklists and charts are completed by the primary health care provider and pass this information on to a focused specialist who then reviews it before having a video conference with the patient and health care provider. The virtual consult specialist provides all connections (including video conferences) and monitors and records all communication. The focused specialist is mandated to ask the consult specialist if there are any questions, comments or concerns at the end of every video conference with the patient. The focused specialist will then determine the course of action. If admission is required, the focused specialist works on deciding the treatment/care plan. Meanwhile, the virtual consult specialist arranges admission by finding a bed at the Focused Centre of Excellence where the focused specialist works.

The consult specialist notifies the transport coordinator to arrange transportation if required. The focused specialist will decide on the treatment/care plan which is either standard care, or custom care and will inform the consult specialist. The standard treatment plan is evidence-based care and provides the focused specialist with a standard template. It is somewhat like a check list with each item to be initialled as care is provided. The custom plan would have all care by the focused specialist recorded on their self-designed detailed treatment/care plan. The consult specialist will review both types of treatment plans checking for inconsistencies, conflicts, omissions or other problems that could result in adverse outcomes.

The treatment plan may incur minor changes in the standard care template but must be in consultation with the virtual consult specialist unless it is considered an emergency. The FS will explain the reason for the change, the advantages and disadvantages. The VCS may make recommendations or indicate agreement or not. Change may also occur to the custom treatment plan but this too must be reviewed by the consult specialist to assure it is the best and safest it can be. The focused specialist would be consulted but is not obliged to comply with any recommendations. The virtual consult specialist also connects a FS to do voluntarily consult with all health care providers, regardless of whether the patient requires admission or not. It will be up to the primary care provider to request a consult. This may occur when nurse practitioners, paramedics or physicians have an unusual case, or the patient is requesting a second opinion.

Benefits of the Health Consultation Centre (H2C)

– The patient will be given a choice of one out of three focused specialists to choose from. The focused specialists may or may not be from different Focused Centres of Excellence.

– It provides mandatory consultation for a patient at a primary care site that has been seen twice for the same problem and is now in for a third time with the issue still unresolved. The virtual consult specialist will be contacted and will arrange a video conference with a focused specialist.

– If transportation is required, the VCS will request a transport coordinator arrange transportation to another site.

– If the primary health care provider requests a consult, the VCS will connect the provider with the required focused specialist.

– The virtual consult specialist (VCS) will consult on the diagnosis and treatment plan provided by the focused specialist and in essence, provide a co-pilot second opinion.

– The VCS will provide a smooth transition for the patient through the health care system.

– The VCS will keep the health care providers up to date on best practices.

– The VCS will in conjunction with the HTC provide a better coordinated inter-city and inter-IQSA RR…scheduled transport system

– The VCS may facilitate physical examination with an FS when required.

- The VCS will coordinate efficient use of all in-patient beds in the province.

– The VCS will standardize electronic medical record formats and storage systems.

– The VCS will review treatment plans and ongoing care in consultation with health care providers. This could be the airline equivalent of a flight plan filed with an air traffic controller. This would be an extra level of safety to assure the treatment plan is adhered to and assure reasons for change are valid.

– The VCS will promote standard care evidence-based best-practice treatment.

– The H2C could be put to additional uses such as tracking antibiotic resistant diseases and contagious viruses.

– Virtual consult specialists at the H2C will track performance indicators through innovative reporting mechanisms.

As noted earlier, physicians are well educated, respected, and trusted. Mandating them to follow standard medical care protocols or medical directives whether evidence based or not, does not give them the flexibility, when necessary, to customize treatment for the best outcome of any particular patient. They should retain the right to treat the patient in the best way they see fit. But this also means that there is a greater chance of an adverse effect. To reduce this chance, a care/treatment plan will be introduced for all patient care. The co-pilot is the virtual consult specialist, and the flight plan is a treatment plan. There are two types of treatment care plans, the standard care and the custom care. All nurse practitioners, paramedics, family physicians/specialist and emergency physicians requesting a consult may result in an FS wanting to admit the patient. In addition, voluntary consults, not concerning admission, may be requested at any time. The paperwork concerning a patient receiving standard evidence-based care will include all steps to be taken. Each step will be followed as described, and initialed as completed. However, if a change is required, contact with a consult specialist is required. Minor changes may be allowed; however larger changes may result in the need for a custom treatment plan to be submitted. Each step will need to be written into a new custom treatment plan This will necessitate considerable additional time for the FS to complete paperwork.

The health care change to an all-specialist system should make staffing the virtual consult centre easier as there will be many more specialists. The virtual consult specialist never comes into contact with the patient. Their function is to assure the best care for the patient. The virtual consult specialist works in the background and is as unobtrusive as possible, not usually evident to the patient even though they are told the video conference is monitored and a second opinion will be given. Each treatment plan will be reviewed by the virtual consult specialist checking for inconsistencies, omissions, and conflicts, especially with prescribed drugs or any other actions that could be performed in a safer way. Any of these discoveries would be brought to the focused specialist's attention as suggestions. This also applies during live video conferencing consults which are monitored for the same reasons, and anytime questions, comments or concerns arise that have not yet been answered during the video conference between the patient and the focused specialist, the virtual consult specialist may make inquires at the end of the conference, after the focused specialist asks the consult specialist if there are any questions, comments or concerns. In the past, second opinions were optional and often proved time consuming. Now it will be mandated as indicated and much faster. This might be best done through texting or a private phone call, so as not to confuse the patient as to who is in charge of their care The focused specialist will then ask the patient any questions the VCS has for the patient. Patients are informed that all conferencing is monitored by another specialist to enable a second opinion. After the video conference is over and any VCS questions have been answered, the patient will be informed by the FS regarding the treatment or whether admission is required.

The virtual consult specialist will monitor and record communication between health care providers and focused specialists, and between patients and FS, and between health care providers at different facilities. Monitoring starts at a primary care facility, when a mandatory consult has been requested during the third visit, after the first two visits did not resolve the health care issue, or if voluntarily requested, or between health care providers at different facilities such as when a focused specialist has a video conference with the staff or patient at a tertiary care hospital.

For patients to be admitted, consultation between the focused specialist, the primary care provider, the patient, and a virtual consult specialist is mandatory. But the option to contact the virtual consult specialist at any time is always there. The current EMR could be used for the IQSA system. By requesting the EMR through the VCS, it will help assure confidentiality and privacy of information.

The virtual consult specialist will try to find a focused specialist to admit patients locally within the originating IQSA RR whenever possible. But because each IQSA RR only has a maximum of three categories of care for Focused Centres of Excellence, this may not always be possible. The odds of finding a bed locally for those that require extended recovery time are much better as every IQSA RR will have tertiary hospitals.

Looking at evidence-based standard care as a refined process is key. Introducing it at the primary care level may be very effective. Every condition will have an evidence-based standard treatment plan available. This should speed up service, reduce unnecessary assessments and tests, and lower costs.

All consults are in conjunction with a focused specialist. The consult specialist would not do this on their own. They would arrange for a focused specialist to have a video conference with the primary care provider and the patient, and then at the end of this conference and on request, the VCS would provide a second opinion. This request is mandatory.

After the consultation, the consult specialist, the focused specialist and the primary care provider will consult among themselves to help the focused specialist determine the course of action. If there is a problem on the diagnosis, the matter is referred to a diagnostic team consisting of a few consulting specialists at the H2C. Their diagnosis is provided to the focused specialist and the VCS. The FS will consider the result of the diagnostic team but is independent to decide the diagnosis and treatment that they will provide. The patient may also request another focused specialist. If a request occurs the patient will be booked another appointment and go through the same procedure again with a different FS but may only do this once and the result may be the same.

The consult specialist at the H2C would have access to a bed registry that would include all beds in the province for Focused Centres of Excellence, tertiary hospitals, long-term care, and others such as hospice, focused living, and retirement homes will be encouraged to participate in the bed registry. They would also have access to a physician registry to enable them to know which three focused physicians are next in line to receive a patient. Another important function is to refer cases where the patient requires transport to the health transport centre where a health transport coordinator will coordinate all patient transfers for those requiring scheduled transportation. Emergencies will still be managed in the same way as they are now with the ambulance system.

When the VCS is contacted, whether it was optional or mandated, it will be their responsibility to assign the proper VCS and FS specialist to the case. Both the VCS and the FS will be the same type of specialist. If possible, the same VCS and focused specialist will provide all care to the patient once admitted by the FS and that care will continue at the tertiary care centre if required. The only exception is if the patient needs the services of a sub-specialist or another type of specialist.

When the consult specialist is contacted, they will always recommend standard evidence-based care. If the focused specialist believes a custom course of treatment may be of greater benefit to the patient, the focused specialist may proceed with the care they feel is best, provided the patient agrees. If not, the focused specialist may go along with the patient's request or the patient may request another focused specialist in which case the patient will be booked for another appointment, but this can only be done once.

The people in charge of developing evidence-based standards of care, clinical practice guidelines, and medical directives must be totally independent, free of lobbyists and those that may try to influence them. Their decisions must be transparent. This also applies to those physicians on the diagnostic team. Creating standardized care pathways is not a new idea.as the following statement in a report from pricewaterhousecoopers indicates (paraphrased) Some countries report standardization is happening in both administrative and clinical areas with administrative standardization moving faster. Netherlands and Germany, are introducing case rate payment systems, that are expected to help lead toward more standardized care pathways. [xxi]

Chapter Highlights

The chapter explains the need to create a Health Consultation Centre (H2C) at all Focused Centres of Excellence and employ a full range of virtual consult specialists that will rotate positions with focused specialists. The diagnostic team which will also be located at the Health Consultation Centre will assist with difficult to diagnose cases and is also responsible for research and development into evidence-based standard care pathways and medical directives. It is anticipated that for every one virtual consult specialist there will be five focused specialists providing hands-on care to patients at the Focused Centres of Excellence.

*Please note: the focused specialist is referred to as the admitting/ attending specialist in some cases. In most cases, the focused specialist provides all care except where a sub-specialist exists at the Focused Centre of Excellence.

Fig. C

Communication Algorithm

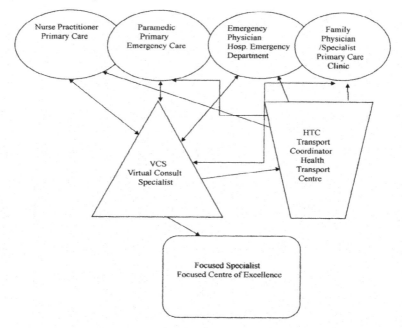

CHAPTER 7

Trends in Health Care

Examining how health care has been evolving over the decades may provide insight into current trends and where we should be heading. Hospital care in the 1930s, 1940s, and 1950s consisted of many smaller community hospitals providing what would have been a broad range of services, hence the name *general* hospital. But as the number of services expanded, beyond what the small community hospitals were capable of providing, many services gradually shifted to larger regional hospitals. Such services were generally newer types of treatment which required large investments in expensive equipment (i.e., CT, MRI, and PET scanners) and/or specially trained technicians and physician specialists.

These larger hospitals, often referred to as regional hospitals, served large areas. Much of the regional hospital space was devoted to typical general hospital work, but gradually more space was devoted to specialized work that no other hospital in their region provided. This was primarily because it was not economically feasible for the smaller community hospitals to have expensive equipment and specialized staff that would sit idle, waiting for patients. At the regional site, equipment and staff could be shared by all patients coming from the smaller community hospitals in the area.

Today we have reached the point again where the number of services has expanded greatly, and some of these are very specialized. With the expansion of such services comes more patients. Patients that there was no medical help for in the past, now have options. This combined with a general increase in patient populations and associated demand for services. The result? We now have many regional hospitals experiencing demands they find difficult to meet. Hospitals are being spread too thin. And so too is their funding. They still provide good care in general and specialized services when possible but access is still questionable at times. This is because of the current way they are structured which means services cannot meet the high demand for care or deliver it at the time it is requested. Pricewaterhousecoopers May 2002 HealthCast Tactics: A Blueprint for the Future, says (paraphrased) Including high-quality, high-margin, high volume services are what leading hospitals are doing.[xxii]

The larger regional hospitals have now reached the point where smaller community hospitals were sometime ago. Now it is the regional sites that cannot provide all the care. That is why they transfer some of their patients out to large provincial centres that may be in other IQSA RRs. There, the hospitals provide care to patients from all points in the province, and sometimes from beyond. These provincial hospitals (as I call them) specialize in care others do not, including the regional hospitals. In some cases, they may provide care in the same field but to a much more intensive degree that a regional hospital can, and because there are so few of them, they are often located some distance away from the patient. The government has a grading system that refers to the level of care provided by some provincial hospitals. Trauma is one, which may be referred to as a level one or level two trauma hospital. A level one trauma centre is the top rated and can accept the most severely injured patients that other hospitals are not equipped to manage. A level two, unlike a level one, is not a teaching or research centre but can provide the same level of care.

Patients are aware that occasionally travel may be necessary in today's system. So, the changes recommended here should not come as a complete surprise. Large regional hospitals, usually one for each IQSA RR, treat a wide variety of conditions, but often sections of them now days are specialized and treat conditions that few other hospitals do. Neither the specialized services nor the general treatment part of these large regional hospitals is able to keep up to demand. There may be many causes. Perhaps demand is higher than anticipated or perhaps funding and staffing issues arise. Many new services have been added to the general section of the hospital that may be spreading resources too thin and the specialized units may not be functioning at optimal levels because they are too small. Developing hospitals that treat a wide variety of conditions makes it difficult to focus and excel in specific areas.

Further refining Focused Centres of Excellence may consist of many possibilities, such as the design of the unit, the purchasing of user-friendly equipment, barcoding patients to prevent errors, the bulk purchasing of supplies and equipment, having physicians onsite 24/7, and reserving physician time for service that only they can provide. All this will increase efficiency. As an example, in one hospital in Manitoba, the surgeon that does hip replacements performs only that part of the surgery that requires his expertise, while a physician assistant opens and closes the patient. The surgeon is kept busy going from one operating room to another. In this way, more work is accomplished in less time.

Big changes in society have spurred significant changes in business. Mass manufacturing has made a tremendous difference in our lives and mass retailing has delivered it to our door. Giant stores such as Walmart and Costco deliver vast quantities of goods. Without them, it would take thousands of mom-and-pop stores to deliver the same volume of goods. Larger populations, the vast array of goods produced, and competition all combine to drive the marketplace in this direction.

Health care cannot be the exception. While the specialization of health care would be a prerequisite for the care of vast numbers of patients, it cannot happen if the facilities and the processes used do not match the desired output. In the days before mass production, there were few goods to be sold and what there was could easily be sold in small general stores. But that is far from the case today.

We can draw an analogy. In the past, there was little that could be done for many medical ailments, so the way health care was delivered matched the options available. The closest equivalent to the mom-and-pop general store would be the small community hospitals of the 1940s, 1950s, and 1960s. These stores provided a limited array of goods with a very high level of personal service. Often, they knew what you wanted before you even asked for it. Bags were filled and delivered to the car or to the home. The manager often knew the customer personally and often lived in the same neighborhood and would extend personal credit when banks would not.

The small community hospitals also provided what we today would say was a limited range of services but was normal at the time, and the doctor at the hospital may also have been your neighbour. The doctors that worked there were often the same family physicians that would make house calls. They got to know you as a person, not just a patient. It was a much closer relationship.

Then things started to change. Slowly the mom-and-pops began fading out and the department store gained ground. The mom-and-pop stores could not compete on price because they could not sell the volume of goods that the department store could, nor could the mom-and-pops offer the same variety of goods. The personal service that we knew fell by the wayside, as we seldom knew or saw the department store manager. He tended not to live in the same neighbourhood and the service was not as personal. Cutbacks in staffing levels per square foot led to an increase profit but also meant we had to find our own way around the store because it was difficult finding assistance.

The closest equivalent in health care to the department store of the 1970s and 1980s is the regional hospital. The regional hospital offered a wider range of services and could provide care to more people. Generally speaking, we did not know the people that worked there, and they knew little about us unless it was written in the patient chart, so it was less personal than the small community hospital. The department store of that era was effective and a good choice at the time, just as the regional hospital was, but neither meet our needs today. Now, the department store is being replaced by big-box superstores. They offer vast amounts of consumer goods but generally in a smaller range with a wider selection in that range. As an example, some stores specialize in, lumber and associated building and home products, some specialize in hobbies and crafts, some clothing, and others business and office supplies, to name a few, and sell to large numbers of people. It is all delivered within a no-frills décor, where they have managed to cut costs, sell for less, and outsell the department store. Costco, for example, does this by selling in bulk.

The closest health care equivalent to the modern big-box superstore of today would be the IQSA system of tomorrow. It will provide vast numbers of patient's high-quality care at lower costs when they need it. This is accomplished through the creation of super-sized Focused Centres of Excellence, highly specialized, that provide care with physicians onsite 24/7. They too would only provide that part of the care where only their expertise is required. Other health care professionals would assist with the work. Because of their size, far fewer units would be needed, possibly only one to three in each category of care in the province.

To meet the need today and in future, health care must be provided on a mass scale with as much standardization as possible. These changes will improve the system so much as to make it unrecognizable. Bringing health care to the patient efficaciously, efficiently, and effectively means including every advantage that the facilities, infrastructure, and staff can provide. That means using it 24/7. Nothing can be allowed to sit idle. The whole system needs to function 24/7, not just parts of it like it is today.

Henry Ford discovered that his assembly line was only as fast as its slowest point. That slowest point is often referred to as a bottleneck. Having a 24-hour emergency department funnel into a hospital that for the most part, only has physicians working during the day, creates a tremendous bottleneck. The best functioning parts of today's system are specialized, and have managed to refine the work process to smooth out or eliminate some of the huge bottlenecks. They often do this by having physicians available for longer hours.

Unfortunately, because they are still only a small part of a general hospital, some of their problems are not theirs alone but are ingrained in the hospital system, often making change difficult. Specialized parts of the hospital depend on departments within the hospital that are backlogged with work causing slowdowns. They have been this way for some time, but the problems have been exacerbated by Covid-19. Megan Ogilvie reports that Paige Taylor White *of the Toronto Star notes* St. Michael's Hospital *Dr.* David Gomez, says the backlog means that (paraphrased) unless we change the way we are doing things needed surgeries won't get done in Ontario [xxiii] Emergency departments can not admit patients because the rest of the hospital is full or the process depends on parts of the hospital that are unable to manage requests because the majority of employees work dayshift.

Stores like Walmart smoothed out some bottlenecks and have done so by going online. Retail stores are evolving into more of a combination retail store and warehouse where goods purchased online any time of day or night can be picked up. If health care is ever to catch up with the way that the Western standard of living is evolving, it too would need to provide services on a very large scale, and do it 24/7.

What drives these changes? Some of the main factors could be population growth, population aging, technology, and economic and social changes in society. Today, both spouses work and more often, both work full time. Going to a 9 to 5 office or clinic for health care is not an affordable option. Many do not have paid sick time. Many have more than one job, especially part-time employees. When a child is sick, the current system often requires that the parent take time off work. The population is growing and with it, the demand for care. Our high standard of living can't be met with solutions that past generations used. But the principal can remain – care for all through public insurance.

We really do need to look around. Modern Western society is full of examples where the processes and equipment used to manage growing demand in industry have seen a shift from small applications to medium to large and now extra-large ones. Double-deck super-jumbo jets carry hundreds of people and super-large cruise ships carry thousands. Manufacturing and warehouse sites (fulfillment centres) are enormous, and the retail world is made up of many box-type superstores bringing mass merchandising to the consumer along with online stores like Amazon. There are no more mom-and-pop general stores. It would take thousands of such stores to now replace these big-box and online stores. Stores like Walmart succeed because they deal with volume. They do things small stores cannot. They manage vast quantities in a global empire; they are open longer; they have lower prices and fast product turnover. Much of this can be applied to health care.

It is a 24/7 world. The internet, smartphones, and a hectic everyday lifestyle all contribute to the need for change. Health care has tried to adapt. In the last decade or two, there was a strong push to staff all emergency departments with emergency physicians 24/7. In the past, many small departments only had physicians on call. Larger emergency departments slowly recognized the need for two main branches of emergency care: emergency care (those that will require admission), and urgent care (those that do not require admission). They thusly created two separate treatment areas. The purpose of this division was to provide faster service to those with urgent-care needs and leave room in emergency. Physicians in the urgent care department often came from the emergency department, which in some cases meant slower urgent care when emergencies were a priority. This combined with the fact that urgent care was seldom provided 24/7 meant it was only a partial answer.

Primary care has seen many attempts at improvement, some with limited success. A few of these included family health networks, family health organizations, family health teams, health care centres, after-hours walk-in clinics, and urgent care centres. None of these were 24/7, and few provided all urgent services required to meet primary emergency care needs (defined as emergency care for those that do not require admission).

We cannot turn back the clock. The pressure is only going to increase. We are in the age of 24/7 communication. Information flows freely. People can shop online 24 hours a day. Society is changing and the expectation is increasingly moving toward being able to do what needs to be done, any time of the day or night.

The public health care system evolved from its private care system roots. For years there was no need to change it. Private care did not work as a system. Each part of private care developed to meet its own internal needs. When the public system came about it took over private care and added public health insurance. Other than that, there was little change for a very long time. But ever so gradually, public care began to realize its new-found potential and started to act a little more like a cohesive system where patients could be transferred between health care facilities with greater ease because it was a single-payer system. Eventually, regional hospitals began to provide newly developing services not feasible with smaller hospitals.

It is interesting to note the evolution of the emergency department. It too was a design that carried over from the days when the system was private. In those days, many family physicians provided suturing of lacerations in the office, and those with fractures might have casts applied in-office as well. Fewer patients were required to go to the emergency department for issues that did not require admission. The downfall of this, was the fact that it was based on the premise that their family doctor's office was *open* and that he did these procedures in the office.

Once government brought in the publicly funded system, it was decided all doctors in Ontario would be paid on a fee-for-service schedule. This added considerable time to the billing process as each procedure was required to match up with a code and submit this to the government for reimbursement. Why was this? Physicians thought of themselves as independent contractors and did not want to be on salary and be considered employees of the public system even though it might have made their lives a little easier. This meant that the faster they worked, the more money they made. Physicians discovered that their wages could increase by eliminating time-consuming treatments. Patients were gradually referred more often to the emergency department if their treatment could not be accomplished in the normal visit allotment time. Suturing and setting fractured bones with casts are indeed two-time consuming procedures. Physicians also saved money by not having to stock supplies or equipment related to such procedures.

The emergency department, once designed more for critical emergencies, now started to treat an increasing number of urgent cases referred by office physicians. Gradually, with limited hours of operation at doctors' offices, the public understood where they had to go to receive the treatment they required and would bypass doctors' offices in those types of situations.

Tracking time is part of any good business. Time is money and this applies to health care in general, and the ways physicians work as well.

Physicians in their office have been doing time monitoring for decades and that is one reason why some patients are referred to the emergency department. Time management is now affecting other types of patients that require more attention, such as patients with multiple chronic conditions. Some physicians now carefully limit their practice and do not accept many of these types of patients.

Changing the way that the emergency department works is part of the solution. Separating emergency patients into the two main branches must continue but the need now is to recognize who is best suited to provide each type of care and where the care should be provided?

Ideally, human resource allocation works on the principal that the person best suited to perform the work does the job. Not the one underqualified or overqualified. Over time, as the changing world of work continues its relentless march, new workers will evolve to meet new demands. Paramedic practitioners are one such kind of worker. Highly specialized, with education and skill to fit into the exact place in the health care system where they are needed. By working in conjunction with nurse practitioners and other health care providers, linked to specialists, we will have a system truly ready to adapt to the 21st century. Retaining emergency physicians for patients that require admission to the hospital or in the new system, Focused Centres of Excellence, would be putting *their* services, knowledge, and skills to maximum use. To use paramedics for primary emergency care (those not requiring admission), would be putting *their* skills and knowledge to maximum use. And to increase the numbers of nurse practitioners and specialists would let the system evolve with technology to match. Much of what paramedics do can apply to primary emergency care, but because paramedics do not currently provide all these services, additional training will be required. Recognizing and providing specialists for both emergency care and primary emergency care is part of the IQSA system, but in this case, one of the specialists is a paramedic. Each of these changes will enhance the patient experience by better matching their needs to the right provider.

In the UK, paramedic training is in levels consistent with care demands. The highest level is a degree program at university. Here in Canada, some paramedics could be trained through a university program to become paramedic practitioners. The additional education could meet the needs of primary emergency care. In the meantime, current paramedics are just shy of the training required to meet all primary emergency care needs. Until that program is in place, some paramedics could be upgraded with a part-time program to meet the future paramedic-practitioner standard.

In turn, this change and all others will contribute to making the system more integrated quality sustainable and accessible (IQSA). If paramedics were to set fractures in casts at primary emergency care centres, they would only do so, as a temporary measure until the patient could be transferred to a specialist for care. This is how it is often done today for a patient arriving at an emergency department. Once the X-ray is taken and a cast applied, the emergency physician makes an appointment for that patient to see an orthopedic specialist.

Health care administrators have worked at trying to reorganize primary care and have created the many models previously mentioned. In all these reorganizations, the changes were done to respond to two main problems: patients requiring primary care, without family physicians and patients needing urgent care called primary emergency care in this book. The new physician provided services sometimes had longer hours and the physicians were paid differently so they could spend more time with patients. The Auditor General indicated there were 17 different type of payment schedules for physicians in 2012

By incorporating many different types of health care providers at the primary care site, they have lessened wait delays for appointments or when traveling to meet with other providers. In this way they have been successful at providing additional primary care, but they have not been able to provide 24/7 primary emergency care, thereby causing many patients to go to the hospital emergency department and overload the facility. In addition, the teams have not been rolled out in sufficient quantities to meet the needs and have various operating hours.

This could be a result of funding and staffing difficulties that were a problem for some family health teams (FHT). Walk-in/after-hours clinics and urgent care centres might have had a much larger impact on the emergency department if they were open 24/7, and provided all primary emergency care needs, but this does not appear to be happening. For system change to happen in a coordinated and comprehensive fashion, one prototype needs to be designed, built, and tested on all pertinent parameters (i.e., efficacy, efficiency etc.). Then the calculation on total provincial cost can be worked out based on the number of units required. This gives a better idea on whether we can afford the prototype proposed, or if a redesign needs to be done.

The emergency department needs to be divided into emergencies requiring admission and those that do not. Naturally, emergencies requiring admission would be best located at a hospital emergency department where the emergency physician specialists can care for the patient, whereas primary emergencies not requiring admission should be strategically located, often located next to an ambulance service station or a nurse practitioner clinic or both.

As health care takes on a coordinated system approach, it will make connections in ways not considered before, and this will be done through the Health Consultation Centre (H2C). All specialists at Focused Centres of Excellence will be connected to all tertiary care centres, primary care clinics, primary emergency care centres, hospital emergency departments, and others. All focused specialties will have matching virtual consult (VCS) specialists to act as co-pilots. A ratio of approximately one VCS specialist to every five focused physician specialists may be a good starting point. The job description for the VCS has not been determined which makes it difficult to pinpoint the exact ratio.

The health consultation centre (H2C) will also be responsible for collaborating with the HTC to arrange transportation when required, collaborating with FS to determine updates to evidence-based care, providing input into standard care template check sheet design, listening to patient interviews, reviewing patient charts, and in future, reviewing treatment and producing video for teaching purposes and more.

While working at creating a coordinated system and improving the process of caring for the patient, the system must evolve to introduce better safety measures. The system is aware of errors occurring but not enough attention is paid to assuring that they are not repeated. In the future, health care may have many more parallels with the airline industry. The airline industry regards accident investigations as a high priority. It is only because of the constant efforts to make travel safe that the industry has expanded. For some people, air travel is so commonplace it feels the same as taking a bus. For air travel to have reached this point, many hard lessons were learned, many that would benefit health care. When a crash occurs, a special investigation team goes to the scene to determine the cause. The team scourers the accident site, reconstructs the aircraft, reviews flight recorders, interviews survivors and witnesses, reviews flight and maintenance logs, and checks on pilot credentials and lifestyle. As a result, many potential flaws in the system are corrected before more tragedy occurs.

In health care, the coroner's office does have a death review committee that in many cases investigates some hospital deaths, but more needs to be done. Medical errors (adverse effects) that do not result in death but have negative outcomes need to be investigated. Some errors may cause death, but most do not. Studying adverse effects and correcting the underlying causes may have a ripple effect, lowering the unexpected death or disability rate across the board.

How do we reduce the number of errors. Unless we are aware of the errors and keep track of the errors it can't be done. A new independent investigative body that might be called the Health Safety Investigation Board. could be created by all IQSA RRs combining resources. It would review cases of non-lethal medical adverse effects to determine what might be done in future to prevent the adverse effects from reoccurring. The investigation would examine all relevant aspects including the patient, hospital, clinic, ambulance or freestanding health unit, the health professionals involved, the regulatory college, the ministry of health, relevant technology, and drugs, and they would review charts, video and audio recordings made by the VCS.

After all relevant questions have been answered and the facts compiled, recommendations can be made. Just as with air transportation accidents, there is seldom one cause of a death or injury. There are usually several contributing factors and that is often the case with non-lethal adverse effects in health care. There is much more that can and should be done to improve safety. After all, advancement without safety is a fallacy. The function of the investigation board is not to find fault, civil or criminal liability, but only to improve the system.

The Ontario government passed a law called "Quality of Care Information Protection Act, 2004." According to the Ministry of Health and Long-Term Care website, the act is designed to encourage health professionals to share information and have open discussions about improving the quality of health care delivered. This includes learning from critical incidents in their organizations that involve the delivery of patient care, without fear that the information will be used against them.

Chapter Highlights

Current and future demand will see a shift to large units running 24/7 with physicians always present and new measures in place to maintain quality and detect the possibility of adverse effects before they happen. Today there are large hospitals and, in the US, large multi hospital corporations. This is good but the health care system needs to go a step further and specialize with large, focused units. Then the process can be streamlined with increased speed and satisfaction. No one wants to be in a hospital but we all want quality work to recover as quickly as possible. Experienced specialized medical staff will assist with this.

CHAPTER 8

Additional Considerations

Bringing health care into the 21st century will be a challenge. The IQSA Health Care System is a long-term goal and may take up to 15 years to implement but short-term thinking leads to short-term solutions, especially when it comes to health care. If the redesign of the system starts as indicated in the timeline we may see relief and improvement in some of the most overburden part of the system in just a few years. To provide care IQSA will need to build facilities. Neither public or private is an instant solution. Some parts of the system will need to be expanded and other parts will need to be eliminated. Some parts will need to be rethought while other parts can remain the same. Taking one step at a time and allowing the system to adapt before moving on may help.

The IQSA Health Care System could start with having one IQSA RR choose the categories of care (max: three) that they would like their three Focused Centres of Excellence to provide. The size of the Focused Centre of Excellence would be a 200, 300, or a 400-bed unit. Consultation with other IQSA RRs may result in some swapping of Focused Centre of Excellence bed size. Then, training would be offered to family physicians to upgrade to specialties with incentives to train for the areas chosen by the IQSA RR in which they are located. This would require a concerted effort among many players that may include the Ministry of Health and Long-Term Care, the IQSA RR, the College of Physicians and Surgeons, and the medical schools and physicians themselves, to name the main ones.

Implementing the IQSA Health Care System will bring health care in line with the standard of living that we are accustomed to. As it stands today, access to health care is in sharp contrast with most other goods and services in Canada. Most do not require lengthy wait periods or provide sub-standard accommodation. All admissions will be for specialized care and will be organized to serve the whole province, with patients arriving from anywhere in the province. This will reduce wait times and will be achieved with the creation of a system of Focused Centres of Excellence. The units will function with well-defined processes that will speed care, quality, efficacy, and efficiency.

The IQSA system still provides care locally for primary care, primary emergency care, emergency care and tertiary care, and locally for those chosen Focused Centres of Excellence specialized services. When appropriate, out-of-hospital patient care (out-patient) will video teleconference with FS going through a VCS at a primary care site. If this will not suffice, then arrangements can be made for the patient to proceed to the Focused Centre of Excellence where the focused specialist can meet with the patient in person or if applicable, the physician can recommend that the patient visit with an assessment team. Assessment teams may be set up in multiple IQSA RRs to meet varying needs. The former northeast LHIN (area 13) had a joint assessment centre (knee and hip) that had an advanced-practice physiotherapist that would help determine the best treatment for patient joint care whether it be surgery, physiotherapy or other treatment. Another that may be feasible is the geriatric assessment centre that helps determine treatment for various geriatric problems. It consists of a clinical nurse specialist, a physiotherapist, an occupational therapist, a dietitian, a social worker, and a resource consultant.

At one time, every hospital attempted to provide every service possible. Then it changed to every regional hospital, and then changed again to every LHIN (Local Health Integration Network). The number of services available has multiplied and the number of patients has grown exponentially. The system now has too much duplication with many small units and not enough attention to full service meaning 24/7. The IQSA system will eliminate small-scale duplication of services and in turn, reduce associated problems such as higher costs, recruitment difficulties, overcrowding, and long waits for care. This may also open the door to new and quicker advances in care.

Today, many areas of the province are trying hard to provide all the services they can because providing care locally is the way it's always been and no one has really looked at a change to large-scale care. The change to the Focused Centres of Excellence system would take a cooperative approach, but as you may have noticed, an element of competition is still possible. Each category of care may have up to three focused units providing that same type of care, although they may be of different sizes. Competition to see which unit has the highest quality and lowest cost as reflected in the lowest 30-day readmission rate or other methods such as patient satisfaction surveys could be part of the competition if this is desired.

Each Focused Centre of Excellence unit will become much larger than current units and will be evenly distributed to each IQSA RR, with one or more units usually at the site of the old regional hospital. Over time the Focused Centre of Excellence may begin to introduce more sub-specialty care. This will bring excellence in care to new heights, especially for patients that had limited options in the past.

Thousands of people have worked countless hours to improve the current health care system. Some improvement has resulted but not enough. The changes that have occurred were done with good intent, but without a plan for the whole system, much of the change to date has only proved beneficial on a small scale and not for the province as a whole. The government, the administrators, the health care providers, and the public all want our system to work. It was more a case of not understanding the choices available. It is not their fault that the system isn't meeting the public's needs. It is the system. Old and outdated and made for a different time and place. Business has evolved but health care has been unable to make meaningful change. Instead, we continuously try to put a square peg in a round hole.

This book presents an option to guide the system in a direction that has not been attempted before. Very little suggested here is totally new, but it is the way the ideas are applied in a comprehensive, coordinated fashion that will make the difference. Change will happen partly because each hospital in the current system has too many moving parts to manage well. Trying to oversee the system will require even more work if it is divided up into many smaller parts such as private for-profit clinics. Accountability may be lost. The answer is larger specialized units resulting in fewer moving parts with local accountability.

The following are a few examples of significant changes that were made in the past, but took far to long to take hold. With a little tweaking the system could benefit from them province wide. The IQSA system is waiting and will lead to amazing results.

Nurse practitioners and paramedics were introduced many decades ago. Nurse practitioners in the 1960s and paramedics in the 1970s. In the case of nurse practitioners, their true potential was not realized until the last 10 to 15 years or so, when a few tweaks to their education have allowed them to fill much needed gaps in the health care system. This has taken them from obscurity to mainstream very quickly. Paramedics also have made huge strides in advancing their education and training and have developed very quickly in the last two decades. Currently, some jurisdictions have met the need for greater education through a degree program in para-medicine. There are many barriers to entry in the primary emergency care field that has slowed progress, but as the transition progresses, paramedics will provide care to many more patients that in past, had to wait until they arrived at a well-equipped emergency department.

Separate units such as the coronary care unit, the burn unit, and others were developed in some hospitals back in the 1970s and 1980s. They were usually located at the regional hospital site. The demand for some of these small, specialized in-patient units was not constant enough to warrant the high cost in maintaining them. Some were dismantled, leaving critical coronary care patients and others in the intensive care unit (ICU), which is a general intensive care unit caring for many types of illness or injury.

The medical transportation system developed multi-patient transfer units in the 1980s. One example included a plane and another a bus. Each was able to carry four or five stretchers. Both were discontinued for various reasons.

Re-applying these ideas in a new and exciting way will make a difference. It will involve a combination of strategic moves and a good understanding of where the components need to go to build the IQSA system. Always looking at the past and adapting for the future with a prudent use of the biggest system cost drivers–this is the IQSA way to go.

Cutting back medical school enrollment in the 1990s was a fiscal restraint measure. Enrollment has since returned to normal levels or slightly exceeded 1990s levels. However, some patients still do not have a family doctor and some specialists have very long wait times. It is becoming increasingly difficult to recruit family physicians in small towns and rural areas. Most of these physicians will indicate that there is not enough support, often no place to refer patients, long hours, and no one to fill in for vacations and time off.

When the health care system went public it no longer allowed corporations to employ physicians exclusively for use by their employees. It was suggested at the time that the new public system could have given each city and town their own OHIP (Ontario Health Insurance) plan billing numbers for physician corresponding to the number of physicians needed in the town, but opposition was too great. Today, once a physician has an OHIP billing number, they can go to work anywhere in the province. It is up to the city or town to entice them. As the small towns lose their doctors to retirement or to the big city, many towns and rural areas now feel the need to offer incentives to compete. Has enough money gone into the system? Can taxpayers really afford to train enough physicians to guarantee everyone a family doctor? How can we guarantee everyone a doctor without knowing where they will work or what type of work they will do? Should funding be cut in other areas of the economy to expand health care? These are all questions that can be argued over. But generally, it can be said that the current system does not seem to be operating as efficiently as it could.

Much work has been done at finding more equitable pay scales for physicians. The change to Focused Centres of Excellence will accelerate this work. Antidotal stories concerning current pay scales are indicating less accountability may be occurring. Confusion on what pay scale applies to which physician is problematic. A report by the Ontario provincial auditor general in 2011-2012 says "Ontario has 17 different kinds of arrangements for family doctors, each with a different payment structure."

To increase accountability, all physicians working at Focused Centres of Excellence would be under one pay scale in the beginning, with a possible change to no more than two pay scales in future. One would be for standard care and one for custom care. Both pay scales would be hourly based to better synchronize with all other health care providers in the IQSA Health Care System.

Part of the answer to our health care problems is not to simply look at health care, but to understand the natural progression that occurs in our society as well. As our knowledge base expands, more specialists are employed to manage the flow and make sense of all this information. This, however, is only part of the picture. Imagine all this information taking the shape of a triangle. In the beginning, information through research is highly concentrated with the researcher. This would be the pinnacle of the triangle. As information is passed on to others, the base of the triangle widens; and as more people acquire the knowledge, the wider it becomes. As research reveals new information, the vertical height of the triangle increases. As the information works its way down from the pinnacle, it becomes filtered. By this I mean less theoretical and more practical. Gradually, the information is pulled down toward the base by those that believe they could put the new information into practical application. In other words, information that was only useful to a few becomes useful to many.

This is an important part of the solution in health care. As researchers develop the information into solutions, it is pulled down by specialists who refine and apply it until it is moves on down to the next level for more general use. In the case of health care, it is paramedics and nurses on the front line that are at the base of the triangle. When the information reaches them, it increases their professional knowledge base. As this occurs, a pressure feedback loop forms forcing the level above to reach higher, to go for the next rung on the ladder, so to speak. It is a type of pull-push action punctuated with periods of inaction when the pressure builds. Pressure at the bottom rung of the ladder has been building and pushing up for a while. The time has come for those above to take a step higher. This same sort of thing happens in business as companies compete to provide a better product or service.

This was happening throughout the 1990s as fewer medical students were choosing family medicine and opting for specialties. Fearing a lack of family physicians to provide primary care, many incentives were developed to entice more medical students to go the family medicine route. This has caused a slowdown in the pressure that was building for family physicians to take that step up the ladder.

It was done with good intention. We were and are still having serious problems in attempting to manage the system the way it was originally designed. Back in the earlier days (1940s, 1950s, and 1960s), there were few specialists. We instead depended on our general practitioners (GPs) for most of our treatment. It was a time when most baby deliveries were done by the family physician, (GP) and when the family physician was trained to remove an appendix. They were taught to be much more self-reliant because they had to be. Training has changed. We cannot go back. The amount of information coming down the pipe is increasing. Medical services such as baby delivery and appendix removal are things generally done by specialists now. Today, we must look at maximizing the use of our health-care human resources. We need specialists and we need primary health care providers, but all will be more specialized.

How can care be improved if family physicians take that step up the ladder and become specialists? It may seem like a paradox, but primary care can improve if all family physicians become specialists. As specialists, all primary care will be directly linked to them. It is all about putting resources to better use. The IQSA health care system will improve care with additional specialists by enabling every patient to receive a second opinion. Others that are trained to provide primary care will include paramedics and nurse practitioners. Nurse practitioner clinics will be strategically located to assure access to primary care including places that have been unable to attract physicians for decades. Primary emergency care is similar to urgent care but differs in two major ways. Urgent care is not provided on a 24/7 basis and it is provided by physicians. All primary emergency care is provided on a 24/7 basis and is provided by paramedics. The primary emergency care centres will be strategically located and will be built adjoining an ambulance service base and a nurse practitioner clinic whenever possible. They too would function 24/7. All primary emergency care centres and primary care clinics are linked virtually to many other specialists through the VCS.

It is not just family physicians that are in short supply. Many specialists, including nurses, nurse practitioners, paramedics, and other health care providers are in short supply also. I believe that the shortage may in part be attributed to the stress involved working in a rudderless health care system that is in a constant state of upheaval and unable to meet the population needs. Changing to the IQSA system will correct this. Reorganizing health human resources will give us a better idea of how many professionals are needed in each category of care. Teaching programs can be directed to increase or decrease admissions as required after allowing for other factors such as turnover, retirement, and migration. A better match of supply to need might make the health professions more appealing to more people. The shift to an open blueprint for the system will relieve anxiety. Everyone will be able to see where the system is going. Discussion on the IQSA Health Care System will provide refinement. The number of primary care clinics led by nurse practitioners and primary emergency care centres staffed by paramedics will need to be calculated on a sliding scale to meet needs as family physicians are trained to become specialists.

Will the change described in the book result in more patients without a family physician or primary care provider? No, nurse practitioners will fill in for family physicians as they transition to become specialists. If primary care requires additional health care providers, those specialists unable to find full-time work will be placed onto waiting lists and during the wait they would practice as a family physician/specialist during the interim. This will help reduce primary care wait times overall. If one of their primary care patients requires care in their specialty, then they are able to continue to provide care. If the patient requires care in another specialty the specialist would contact the VCS to refer the patient to another specialist. Some large American cities (LA) have had long-term difficulty providing sufficient numbers of general practitioners (family physicians) for primary care but they have found solutions by having specialists provide primary care as well.

Here are a few benefits to having an all-specialist system:

* The health care system (IQSA) will benefit by being better able to track information on the type of specialists required in the system and all patients will benefit from being able to access a specialist when required.

* The system will not lose highly trained specialists because they are unable to find full-time work immediately.

* The IQSA system will be better able to estimate the wait time required for full time-specialist positions, possibly enticing more specialists to wait rather than leave.

* The system will continue to pay primary care rates to family/ specialists unless specialist care is provided.

* This approach may allow family/specialists to work in areas where the volume of patients in their specialty is not high enough to support the chosen specialty field of work for all full time.

* The shortage of primary care providers is supplemented short term by family/specialists.

* Patients receive primary care and possibly specialist care all from the same physician.

* Some specialists may prefer the family/specialist blended system and remain family/specialists.

* The system will be able to improve the time from referral to treatment and be able to care for more patients.

* The system will be able to improve the process of care at the Focused Centres of Excellence.

So, with the "all-specialist system," we will have many more specialists. The question becomes what does the system do with so many? We can improve quality and make it safer. Safety is a big factor and will be integral in the shift to a 21st century all-specialist health care system as standard.

Maybe we can again return to the airline industry for more inspiration. Over the years, prior to Covid, the number of people that flew had grown immensely and yet the safety record improved. How can we adapt the airline industry focus on safety to health care? Five elements may be applied to health care as follows:

1. Pilots file a fight plan; this would be equivalent to a treatment plan filed by the focused specialist after consultation with the patient and consult specialist.

2. Pilots have a checklist; the consult specialist will have all health care providers sign off on all procedures in the treatment plan as the work proceeds (a type of checklist for health care). Access to patient charts is limited to information regarding current admission and must be requested from the VCS. For complete chart access a request must be made to the consult specialist. The only person with access to all files all the time would be the consult specialist.

3. Every commercial plane carries two pilots; the focused specialist is the admitting/attending physician and would hold a

position similar to that of the plane's captain. The virtual consult specialist (VCS), would be first officer or co-pilot.

4. All links are recorded just as information is on a black box in an airplane. IQSA needs investigative tools to determine where improvements to the system could be made.

5. Every airplane is tracked by the air traffic controller that has a big role in making sure the system is coordinated and safe. This is done in the IQSA system by the VHC (virtual health consultant) at the H2C (health consultation centre) which along with the HTC (health transport centre) coordinate the system.

The FS (the pilot) will decide the treatment (flight plan) by choosing a custom plan or going with the standard evidence-based plan. If evidence-based standard care is chosen the consult specialist will send the forms that include medical directives and protocols for the focused specialist to follow and sign off as steps are completed. If a custom treatment is chosen, the focused specialist would be responsible for drawing up the treatment plan and sending it to the VCS for review. Either of these plans would be the medical equivalent to a flight plan but in much more detail. All treatment plans would require a signature or password code as the work is carried out to indicate completion. All that provide care must sign as completed. Delays in charting may occur during emergencies.

The new treatment plans will integrate time allotment, or as it is referred to in some circles, book time. This is the average time taken by the many health care providers to perform a given task and would apply to all health care providers, including physicians. A time allotment guide would be attached to every step on the treatment plan. The allotment time guide would be developed by those that develop the evidence-based standard care plans. This would take into account a review of the facility the care would be provided in. It would be done this way to get a better understanding of the time required to go from location A to location B and not just the time taken to provide the care. Walking time in many of today's large hospitals can be considerable. Custom care plans would have tentative time allotment developed by the specialist designing the care plan. Care provider time allotment for standard care could be defined as the average time a job requires. The reason? To increase safety. We are all very pressed for time and sometimes we are pushed too hard, causing errors. One cause of error in health care is having too many tasks to do in too little time. Adequate time will therefore be allotted. If additional time beyond the allotted time is required, the reason must be documented. If new technology or techniques decrease or increase task times, this too is taken into account. While no solution is foolproof, a general guide is needed. Having an allotment time may allow some to slow down but others may have to speed up. Overall, a better understanding of productivity may result.

All patients that require admission to a hospital would require the health care provider to contact a consult specialist (the co-pilot) who would then contact a focused specialist at a Focused Centre of Excellence. The FS (pilot) will create the treatment plan (flight plan) in consultation with the VCS (co-pilot). The plan will be evidence-based standard care or custom care. When a consult is requested, the patient's chart containing all pertinent information, such as vital signs, age, date of birth, address, chief complaint, allergies, and current prescribed medications, as well as the reason for the consult, must be completed and ready for transmission to the consult specialist who will add the patient's history, if required and on file, and then forward this to the focused specialist.

We have a system that comes close to this in a number of ways. It is called EMS (emergency medical services). The system was designed for the paramedic (the pilot) to follow medical directives and protocols, (flight plan), all evidence based, but in cases that need clarification or a deviation from those protocols, the paramedic may contact a physician (co-pilot) to request a change. If the change was deemed beneficial it could be granted by the physician.

The creation of two levels of paramedics has led to some communities not receiving the same level of emergency care as others. The ministry designates which communities will have ACP (advanced-care paramedics) and which will have PCP (primary care paramedics) care but communities are beginning to have more say in this. In some cases, the advanced-care paramedic works alone on a first-response vehicle that does not transport patients. This provided a wider advance-care coverage area but opened the door to adverse effects that were less common than when two equally trained paramedics worked together. Advance care paramedics were encouraged to contact an emergency physician if the need arose. However, this happened only in rare cases (emergency physicians are very busy). The informal type of consulting between same level paramedics that went on in bygone days mostly fell by the wayside. But change has started to happen, thanks to technology, some ACP paramedics are able to consult with other ACPs. Usually, it is done through texting. This valuable second opinion has at times eliminated errors that may have been detrimental to the patient. This should be standard practice for all.

The airline industry uses a pilot and co-pilot for safety reasons. With modern technology, one pilot could do what is needed. Both are trained to equal knowledge and skill level but they often vary in level of experience. This allows either one to interject with relevant substantive dialogue and second opinions. Sometimes major missteps are avoided through this type of team approach. Once a flight plan is filed, it is up to both the pilot and the co-pilot to follow it.

Paramedics provide care to the patient through a treatment plan consisting of protocols and medical directives. This might be considered similar to a flight plan followed by a pilot. Many paramedics carry a reference guide in the form of an abbreviated pocketbook containing all protocols and medical directives that they have and, although it is not mandatory, personal experience tells me that many paramedics consult this reference guide as needed. Even experienced paramedics do this because of the ever-changing nature of health care. As research is carried out, updates are applied and often, changes occur on a yearly basis. Without referencing, we rely on our memories and with so many changes occurring yearly, this becomes problematic. Referencing should be mandatory when time permits. Although use of the consult specialist in this book has not been explored for EMS paramedic services, it may be possible to tie the EMS paramedic service into the medical consultation system through the consult specialist for added safety.

So how would this system lend itself to making a safer system overall? Physicians may accept an equally trained and active co-pilot to reduce adverse effects. Potential diagnostic and treatment problems may be discovered before they are employed. To increase safety the future process of communication will be highly structured. When a primary care provider believes, a patient may need to see a specialist, the wheels are put into motion.

The electronic medical record (EMR) data storage system will include all past data, only as time and money become available to enter it. Only select history data at start-up will be included. This is to prevent the high cost associated with entering all past data from derailing the plan moving forward. Most data will be from the system start-up date. New data entered could be done by the nursing staff, focused specialists or other health care providers, as required. The system will be advanced over the current one in that all consult specialists' video and audio recordings will be included and new chart information may be entered by keyboard or in video or audio format, with subtext to prevent misunderstanding. All entries would be reviewed by the consult specialist daily. Nurses and other staff may enter updates on patient condition daily including any concerns or comments onto the electronic chart for review by the focused specialist and consulting specialist daily or as required.

Health care video conferencing is not new. An example is a walk-in clinic in Sudbury and other sites called the "Good Doctor" (www.good-doctors.ca). It has a registered practical nurse in attendance. The nurse assists while the patient video conferences with the physician in another city. The nurse can do minor tests and connect the patient to an electronic stethoscope, otoscope, etc. that allows the physician to do some examination that they can see on a monitor.

Chapter Highlights

All 14 IQSA RRs will work together to assure that each IQSA RR has three Focused Centres of Excellence providing care in a maximum of three categories of care. The Focused Centres of Excellence size would start off as one of each bed size, 200, 300, or 400 in each IQSA RR during the original design phase, but then an IQSA RR may swap out a size with another IQSA RR willing to do so. Each IQSA RR will, however, maintain three Focused Centres of Excellence. Any beds not designated Focused Centre of Excellence beds will be retained as tertiary care beds.

CHAPTER 9

Technology in Health Care

Technology will keep on progressing and improving care, but think about it for a minute. Technology can be very expensive. How can we compensate for this? The only way to optimize the investment is by getting maximum use out of every piece of technology. The initial high cost to purchase the equipment is more than made up for by the fact the technology can run 24/7 without overtime pay, getting tired, needing holidays, or requiring any kind of benefits. As long as we use the equipment as much as possible, it is a huge benefit. This will be done by making sure that everyone that needs the technology has access to it. With the new IQSA system they will. And this will be possible in part by each IQSA RR area specializing in the type of care they provide and doing it 24/7.

Technology in health care is amazing and it is only going to get better. In fact, it is only because of technology that the IQSA system can come about. Video conferencing is commonplace now and needs to be brought into the mainstream of health care. Today's experimental long-distance remote surgery will become commonplace in the future and the IQSA system is well positioned to take advantage of this innovation. Soon microelectronics will enable development of new mechanical organs and biotechnology will grow new ones. These advances and the ways they are delivered can extend our lives while we still remain in good overall health. Video conferencing, texting or emailing your health care provider will become normal and in fact, it is occurring now in some jurisdictions. Soon this will make electronic prescriptions standard. Advances in nanotechnology will create microscopic robots that fight infections at their level. Once injected, they may be remotely controlled or pre-programmed to do their job. They might also be used in advanced surgery. Much is changing and coming down the pipe.

The change in technology means paramedics have been able to expand care using equipment that is fast and portable and can be brought into the home or anywhere else for that matter. This includes ECG machines, defibrillators, cardiac pacemakers, automatic blood pressure machines, blood oxygen level sensors, carbon dioxide level sensors, blood glucose monitors, CPAP positive pressure machines, suction units, mini blood analyzers, ventilators, and more. New machines have revolutionized the way care is provided.

Hospitals are no different. Now they are able to visualize the body in ways we only dreamed of not long ago. As technology advances, patients can do more for themselves in the home, too. Through self-care, patients can check their blood glucose levels, heart rate, blood pressure, and take an ECG, and some kidney disease patients can perform dialysis at home. This is in addition to people that are on home oxygen or are connected to pumps for drug injection or that have other specialized equipment that was not available years ago.

As technology improves it will greatly help to reduce the need for a hospital stay. With more care being delivered at home, caution must be taken in the design of equipment. Too many types of medical equipment are unnecessarily complicated and difficult to use. Many of these devices may in future be used by the patient directly, although the equipment may not have been designed for use by unlicensed users. Redesigning the equipment for home use will make it safer.

As health care moves forward and all health care providers become specialists, it may be discovered that more of the equipment used becomes specialized also. An example might be X-ray equipment. At one time only hospitals had X-ray equipment and it had limited or restricted use by specially trained X-ray technicians. Today X-ray departments are found both inside and outside of hospitals and provide a large range of services for many conditions and purposes. Today, dentists have specialized X-ray machines in their offices, customized for their use and these days, it is often used by non-dentists trained in X-ray operation.

Maybe the future will see more technology developed for additional specialized uses with very limited conditions and purposes. Teaching people to use this equipment would require much less training because of the limited range of equipment use. Provided, of course, that the equipment can be designed to function effectively and safely. This type of limited use should be promoted.

If primary emergency care centre paramedics were able to provide digital imaging for long-bone fractures with either X-rays or ultrasound, they would move closer to the mandate of paramedics being able to look after all primary emergency patients that do not require admission. Paramedics have started using ultrasound as noted The County of Renfrew Ontario Canada, Paramedics use ultrasound, (exact purpose not specified) the following is paraphrased, Paramedics in the area just completed a course in ultra sound after a rigorous education curriculum and will be able to enhance patient care, safety and time to diagnosis. [xxiv]Ultrasound images or x-rays used to determine fractures could, if desired, be sent electronically to a radiologist for rapid interpretation. If the radiologist report finds a fracture, a cast could be placed on the patient by a paramedic prior to transport to the orthopedic specialist at a Focused Centre of Excellence.

Paramedics have experience in applying immobilization devices that are often used on patients with fractures caused from falls, car accidents etc. and they will manage this change well.

As technology develops it is not unusual that people other than the original licensed user begin to use it. An example might be the use of defibrillators once only used in hospitals by physicians. This equipment is now commonly found and used by the lay person most anywhere. Microwaves once only used in industry by trained technicians can be found in nearly every kitchen today.

Allowing paramedics to use X-rays or ultrasound at primary emergency care centres exclusively for long-bone fractures would bring the centre more in line with its mandate of providing care to all those that do not require admission. I envision it operating one of two ways. One is to have a video link to X-ray technicians wherever they may be. The paramedic would prepare the patient for the X-ray following the technician's orders. This would be confirmed by the X-ray technician through a series of cameras in the room able to capture the positioning of the patient and the required X-ray machine setting. After this has been confirmed and the room is vacated (except of course for the patient), the technician would remotely take the X-ray and send it for interpretation.

If simplified use of the current X-ray equipment was needed, a new type of machine could be developed for x-raying of limbs at the primary emergency care centre. The new design of the digital x-ray machine would have it somewhat resembling a CT scanner, but with a much smaller donut that allows for the placement of the limb to be scanned. Rather than the patient sliding into the machine, only an arm or leg would go into it. The limb would remain stationary as the machine spins and moves up the limb, taking pictures at the appropriate location and angle. The machine could be operated remotely by an X-ray technician or simplified controls would allow for a short instruction course for paramedics at the primary emergency centre.

This in no way replaces the wide range of training that an X-ray technician developed over years in college. A trained X-ray or ultrasound technician is qualified to take images of any part of the anatomy or to do many other types of procedures requiring X-rays, whereas paramedics or others would use X-rays machines only for imaging fractures of the limbs. Many physicians were not taught ultrasound use at medical school, but are now using ultrasound in the emergency department on a regular basis after being given a short training course. A short course for paramedics working at the primary emergency care centres would make X-rays very useful. As noted, the X-ray image that the paramedic takes would be interpreted by a radiologist. The IQSA system would provide an increase in the number of specialists and in particular, radiologists that may make it possible for the results of the X-ray to be returned within 10 to 15 minutes. If it is determined that there is a fracture, the paramedic would apply a temporary cast and call the VCS for referral to a specialist. Additional X-rays could be ordered by the specialists at the Focused Centre of Excellence if required.

Many of the ideas for structural change to health care are possible because of the advances in technology. Local primary emergency care centres staffed 24/7 with paramedics are linked through technology to the very best specialists in their field. This will begin to reverse the trend toward falling service levels in an age of rising demand.

Primary emergency centres are one way to offset rising demand in hospital emergency departments, but another would be E-STAT centres. These are a combination ambulance station and primary emergency centre. Ideally, they would also include a 24/7 nurse practitioner clinic. The E-STAT centres would be as plentiful as ambulance stations at a minimum, and like an ambulance station, will provide rapid care 24/7 which is so important in any emergency. This would allow emergency departments at hospitals to return to what many years ago was their main function, to look after those that require admission.

Many people fear change but if the benefits are explained first, people may be more receptive to it.

Change is constant and we cannot stop it, but we can plan for it and guide it in the direction that is most beneficial. Planned change that allows for input from stakeholders has the best chance of success. Change will happen but if change is not planned, it is not guided to the desired end result.

Improvements based on technologies can be very expensive. To justify the expense, the technology must not be allowed to sit idle. When technology is of benefit to a large number of patients, it becomes economically viable and at the same time helps to speed the perfection of the skills needed by the teams providing the service. This is the IQSA system.

Generally speaking, in a free market economy, mass production lowers costs. The more often an item is produced, the greater the reduction in cost per unit. This metric is harder to achieve in health care, but it is not impossible. What we need to do is take some lessons from the manufacturing sector. By this I mean that improvements in processes and technology that result in higher output do not necessarily result in higher wages, but even if they did, the increase should not exceed the gains made through technology. The current approach seems to revolve around controlling costs by preventing the system from expanding to meet our needs. But this means caring for fewer patients as costs rise, creating long wait times. The answer is to increase the use of technology and create better processes that contribute to faster treatment. By providing the right care, at the right time, in the right place, by the right provider could be referred to as the right process. The IQSA system works hard at doing this. The IQSA Health Care System process is designed for large numbers of patients. The current system uses large hospitals, but has few patients in any one category of care and all are demanding resources. The IQSA system uses large special-ized focused units called Focused Centres of Excellence. A smooth pro-cess that concentrates on volume would not be possible for so few patients. Health care providers must not be under qualified or overqualified. The jobs themselves have to be re-evaluated to decide what work should be done by whom. The IQSA Health Care System meets the need with current professionals trained with additional skills to the exact needs of the process in the IQSA Health Care System.

Additional safety and coordination are what the virtual consultation specialist (VCS) is about. They are composed of many types of consult spe-cialists. From the paramedic-led primary emergency care centres to the nurse practitioner-led clinics to the Focused Centres of Excellence. All of these and more will consult "virtually" with the FS through the VCS as noted in previous chapters, thereby making full use of existing technologies.

Longer waits for everything from doctor's office appointment to hos-pital admissions have slowed the system. All these may be the result of many factors such as higher demand, fewer beds, fewer staff, and less fiscal resources per capita.

Chapter Highlights

Technology is a must if we are to improve the health care sector. Technological advances from other sectors of health care or other sectors of society may be molded to benefit additional health care sectors. Ford cre-ated the assembly line providing us with a way of matching high demand with quality at an affordable price. What can health care take away from this? It shows the need for a process. The process must be documented so it can be repeated over and over. The airline industry has provided us with methods for matching high demand without compromising safety. Check lists and equally trained pilots in the cockpit help to provide redundancy, and consults for critical decision making. Combining these attributes whenever possible can turn around the health care sector. New technology has the ability to change the way health care is provided making it faster, less costly and more effective, but it may also make it safer which is a big part of the change. All these changes to improve safety will supplement continuous medical education of which simulator practice is a part.

CHAPTER 10

The Transportation Network

All patients admitted for care will be admitted to a Focused Centre of Excellence. This will provide the finest health care when you need it, but the finest may not be in your town. The IQSA system will take you to the finest no matter where you live in Ontario. This is the evolution of health care. Physician specialists will be present at all times, providing what is anticipated to be standard evidence-based care, for the majority of cases. Doing this will require a superior transportation network. The health care system needs to develop a transportation network just as the education system has. A school bus assures every student of an education, but the education system as a whole sometimes goes far beyond this, assuring that the education is offered in the language and religion of choice. This idea of specialization for students now includes some high schools that specialize in programs such as theatre arts or technology, etc. School buses take students to these schools, bypassing closer schools.

A new transportation system will do for health care what the school bus system did for public education. Make the best available to everyone. The equivalent of allowing access to specialized programs for students will now be applied to health care, providing access to specialized care for all patients at Focused Centres of Excellence. These highly specialized services will be dependent on a good transportation network because the specialized programs will require a larger catchment area, and patients may have to travel longer distances to access care.

For those patients requiring transportation, a new inter-city and inter-IQSA Referral Region provincial health care transportation system made up of custom designed buses will assure every patient excellent health care in the specialty that they require. The inter-IQSA RR is sometimes referred to as just regional for simplification reasons. The inter-city bus only travels within one region whereas the inter-regional bus travels between regions. The operation of the provincial service will be coordinated by the Health Transport Centre (HTC) and in the future, train and plane transportation may also play a part.

To assure focused excellence in health care, the new system will now go beyond providing health care as we know it. All patient care will be highly specialized care for each patient regardless of where the patient lives. From the specialized type of care given at primary care, primary emergency care centres, and emergency departments to the care in Focused Centres of Excellence to tertiary hospital care with staff that have the knowledge, skills, tools, and engineered processes in place 24/7. All focused units will be specifically designed for the type of condition the patient may have and will be available at the time they require it. No longer will a patient's treatment be put off until after the weekend or the holidays or until the day shift comes in. The system will be ready at all times, changing the dynamics of care, saving lives, time, and dollars.

The point is, long-distance travel is commonplace for Canadians. This is a vast country and today it is not uncommon for people to travel across the country or out of the country on vacation or on business. Some patients may therefore prefer to arrange their own transportation to the Focused Centre of Excellence, but for those that prefer not to, the inter-city and inter- regional transport system is needed. This need is not new.

The current system in Ontario frequently requires patients to travel for care. Usually, it is within their region coverage area to the regional (lead) hospital, and sometimes beyond that to another region for specialized care. Today these patients will often supply their own transportation but for those requiring it, they may use the ambulance system even though it was not designed for transfer transport, although some EMS services do have vehicles designed for this purpose. The future will see inter- regional travel become more commonplace. It will be a well-coordinated system moving far greater numbers of patients and at much greater efficiency.

A transportation system has always been part of the health care system but it was designed for emergencies. Today, ambulance paramedics often do more than emergencies. The IQSA Health Care System will have a scheduled Health Transport Network to complement the emergency transportation system (911). But it will be a separate entity. In some localities, there are private companies that provide patient transfers. These companies often purchase used ambulances and employ recent paramedic college graduates. The public ambulance service, which is generally municipality run in Ontario, is known as the emergency medical system (EMS) and may also provide transfers. Some of these are emergency transfers and are justified in this use, but others are not emergencies and would be well suited to a scheduled transport system. The non-emergency transfers are not the best use for emergency ambulances, but in places where they do those types of transfers, there is often no alternative. Neither of these services (public or private) provide a scheduled patient transfer service.

The IQSA Health Care System will provide the patient with the most appropriate conveyance. The 911 emergency ambulance system will remain the same. Only the non-emergency system will change. Depending on the distance, the IQSA transfer service may use fixed-wing aircraft on occasion but mostly it will be by scheduled bus service. Private transfer companies, when available, may fill the void when the patient must travel between a health care facility and the local scheduled bus terminal. The terminals are needed so that the patient may wait in warmth and comfort in a holding room especially in the winter. Because the patient will be able to access the system much sooner, most patients will not be at a hospital when the decision has been made for a transfer. Having them proceed to a separate bus terminal, one not located at a hospital would be best at preventing overcrowding.

Route example

A non-emergency patient in Sault Ste. Marie needs to go to Sudbury for specialized heart care. The transportation is arranged through the health transport centre. The VCS will contact a transport coordinator at the HTC. The patient is first transported to the local transport terminal holding room. This may be provided by a private service if available, or through the local ambulance service that may or may not have a specialized vehicle for this purpose. Here the patient awaits the scheduled inter-city bus service to Sudbury. These highway-type coaches would be a specialty bus capable of accommodating stretchers. These buses do not leave the region. Another regional bus transfers patients between regions.

Once in Sudbury, the treatment could begin. If transportation to a Focused Centre of Excellence outside the region is required, the patient would be transported to the inter-regional transport terminal (holding room) to await the inter- regional bus. Each region would have only one transport terminal for inter- regional transfers but would have many more terminals for inter-city transfers within the IQSA RR.

Fig D

Health Transport System Example

The patient needs to go from Sault St. Marie to the Barrie Focused Centre of Excellence.
Note: The small transfer vehicle only travels between the patient location and the one terminal located in each city. The patient may proceed to the terminal on their own or may be picked up at a local tertiary hospital, primary care site, primary emergency care site, emergency department, family/specialist site, or the patient's home.
The inter-city bus travels between the city terminals in one region only. Each city in the region will have one terminal. One of the city terminals in each region will have a dual purpose and be designated as an inter-city terminal and inter-regional terminal. The inter-regional terminal will often be near the old regional hospital site.

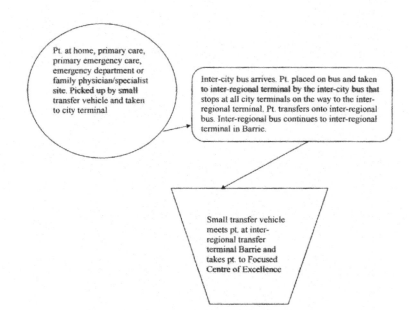

The need to go beyond emergency transportation and provide a scheduled transfer network is long-awaited in the current system. This need only increases with the IQSA RR system as specialized care at Focused Centres of Excellence could be situated anywhere in the province, and some patients will be too ill or unable to travel by private car.

The current health transport system is fractured. Each segment (emergencies, short-distance transfers and long-distance transfers) works in isolation. Good systems are out there in the business world and they could be examples for the health care transport network. One is FedEx. This company delivers parcels worldwide. Long distances are covered by air or tractor trailer, whichever is more practical and quicker. Parcels are delivered to a city terminal and carefully transferred to smaller trucks to deliver parcels locally to their final destination. If another contractor were to provide service at any stage in the transportation of the parcel, careful coordination to prevent a backup of undelivered goods would be required. An important Fed Ex service option is delivery within 24 hours anywhere in the world.

As more Focused Centres of Excellence are created, there will be an exponential increase in the number of patients needing to travel. This in turn will create a need for a superior scheduled transport system to bring patients to and from these Focused Centres from all over Ontario. Most will be travelling long distances for specialized treatment not available in their local IQSA RR area. Emergencies will still travel by ambulance with some requiring emergency air transport because of condition, distance, or geographic isolation. These types of patients will be stabilized at an emergency department and then transported by ambulance (land or air) to the Focused Centre of Excellence in the same way as today.

This is all possible as transportation will no longer be a barrier to care in the IQSA system. Today, patients can be moved around the system very quickly by air or by land ambulances when requiring emergency care, but this is done on a small scale. The future will require a large-scale scheduled network of transportation with the best suited being a bus transfer system, but a rail system (Budd car) might also work in some places.

Using emergency vehicles (ambulances) with paramedics to provide (non- emergency) transfers is equivalent to going to the hospital emergency department for a cold. This practice is a carryover from bygone days when the Emergency Medical System (EMS paramedic ambulances) concentrated on emergencies, fitting in transfers whenever they could. This was possible back in the day because few patients were transferred for care.

In the 1940s and 1950s an ambulance was considered necessary only after a serious accident. This concept gradually changed to include patients that were seriously ill. But you must remember that patients with serious illnesses did not live long in those days so these patients made up a small portion of the required transport. Because of the small number of cases, this usually did not interfere with the ambulance responding to emergencies. Today, we have many chronic and non-emergency patients that require transportation weekly or more often, and the numbers are increasing exponentially. One example might be patients that need dialysis weekly at a tertiary care hospital.

Many different approaches have been tried to manage this significant change. In the beginning it was left to the local ambulance service to provide for all emergencies as well as transfers. Over time it was found that too many ambulances were doing transfers, delaying response to emergency calls, so dedicated crews were created to do the routine (non-urgent) transfers. At first it was the standard two paramedics (one crew) in an ambulance doing emergency calls as well as non-emergency calls, often referred to as transfers. The emergency lights were left on the vehicle and the crew would be diverted from the transfer to an emergency if they were the closest, or if no other ambulances were available.

This defeated the purpose of having a transfer vehicle. Consequently, the emergency lights were removed to prevent the ambulance from being diverted to an emergency. This solved that problem but there were many others. Call volumes for patient transfers continued to increase. From there it was decided that rather than removing the emergency lights from more ambulances so they could be used strictly for transfers, a switch to a bus-type vehicle that could hold many patients would be more practical. This also had another benefit: one paramedic could look after more patients in the back of the vehicle as well. The bus-type vehicle at that time was only used on short-haul routes between hospitals in the same city. This most often happened when a patient required a test on a machine that their hospital did not have.

Problems arose with the bus idea when transport staff (paramedics) tried to keep up with calls coming in from many hospital sites at the same time. This was not a problem before the bus integration as they would just send out more ambulances. To correct for this, the bus was put on a schedule. Various hospitals would no longer be calling at the same time, demanding service. They would know in advance when they could expect service. This scheduled service was not as successful as was hoped for because patients were not always ready when the bus arrived. It could be the patient who was not ready, or the escort, or the paperwork was not done. These delays left some patients on the bus for an hour or more for what should have been a five-minute drive (less than one kilometer) to the next hospital.

When the ambulance service (EMS) could no longer keep up with the volume of transfers, the province started to look the other way as private services began to fill the void. These were cost effective, but many complaints were raised about some private company transfer services and the province has, at times questioned the strategy.

While some of these experimental transfer strategies were occurring, Ontario proceeded with the downloading of EMS to the municipalities. This meant that municipalities were now required to provide ambulances to all emergency calls. The municipalities assumed the role of providing ambulance services and provided good emergency response, but felt it was not their responsibility to provide transfer services, especially for those returning home from outside of their municipality. Privately owned services were thus indirectly encouraged. The latest twist in this dilemma has seen the province providing additional funds to the municipalities to once again provide transfers using vehicles without emergency lights.

Many attempts have been made to rectify transportation problems and there has been limited success where private transfer services exist. The new IQSA system will further reduce the use of emergency vehicles for non-emergency use. The ongoing problem needs to be resolved as the current and future health care system will have an increasing dependence on transfers. The IQSA Health Care System is well organized according to illness or injury, and it will have patients receiving the best care possible in specialized focused units. But such care will often be located some distance from their residences. Transporting patients' long distances for specialized treatment has been going on for some time, but on a limited scale. This happens for various reasons, usually having to do with the expertise, equipment or a bed not being available locally.

Requiring care at a Focused Centre of Excellence may be the next step in care for patients at primary emergency care centres, hospital emergency department, primary care centres, and family/specialist physician offices. If people need emergency care before being admitted, they will be transferred by ambulance to the closest hospital emergency department to be stabilized before transfer to a focused care unit which in many cases may require an ambulance Please note, in the current system the closest emergency department may not be able to provide the most appropriate care, and so some emergency departments may be bypassed in favour of those best able to manage the condition. One example of this is a patient having a stroke. This condition requires taking the patient to a designated site that has a CT scanner which is necessary for treatment of this condition.

Providing the best care possible at Focused Centres of Excellence is dependent on many factors. One of these factors is volume. Higher volumes may lead to improved treatment experience. New types of treatment may be developed and refined at a faster pace. The high volume treated at Focused Centres of Excellence is essential for future IQSA care. Specialization in health care will allow health care professionals to excel and to benefit large numbers of patients. It is only through 24/7 service that patients can be cared for when their need arises. Not just a portion of their care, but all the care they require including physician care. It is only through a totally integrated system, including transportation, that the system can be optimized thereby providing the very best in all it offers. Canada can be the world leader; it is attainable, but it will take work. If we all pull in the same direction, the job will not seem so hard.

The IQSA health system design will be highly dependent on the patient transport system. A look at others in the transportation industry may help assist the design of the health transport system. Let's go back to FedEx, which is a very successful company. Its business model may help us out here.

It could be said that the four main factors that need consideration in the FedEx case are volume, speed, distance, and cost. What is the volume, how quickly must it get there, how far does it have to go, and at what cost? First you might notice that the customer is given an option. How quickly do they want the shipment to get there and what are they willing to pay for that delivery? The faster you want it to arrive the more you will pay. FedEx calls this "express" delivery; the health system calls it an "emergency" and the cost to move a patient by ambulance, land or air is very expensive compared to a scheduled service. How does FedEx handle the express delivery? This depends on the distance the parcel must travel. The formula that Fed Ex uses is not known. However, we can guesstimate that long distances would go by air but it would need to be more closely defined. It may be that anything taking over five hours by land would be considered long distance and depending on the expected time frame may go by airplane; medium distances (up to five hours) would move by tractor trailer; and local deliveries within the city that are defined as within two or three hours would be completed by smaller delivery vans. It is done this way because it is the most economical and efficient and fits within the design parameters.

It would not make sense to send many small vans on the road to the next city when you could send one tractor trailer, or likewise have a large tractor trailer try to make deliveries to a house.

To apply these principals to a patient transfer system means we need to recognize the major factors of volume, speed, distance, and cost. The emergency dispatch system for ambulances works well. This encompasses emergency calls as well as emergency transfers. The patient volume per call is low, usually one patient at a time, the speed is assisted with lights and siren, the distance is usually short, and the cost is high. They do this with the FedEx equivalent of the small van-type vehicle or, if the patient is not accessible by road, then a helicopter is called in.

The patient transfer system in Ontario is currently provided by the municipal ambulance service and private company transfer vehicles similar to ambulances, but without emergency lights. This system is not providing proper utilization. The factors of volume, speed, distance, and cost must be considered in patient transfer. Currently, the transfer volume is high, speed equals the posted maximum, the distance may be long, and the cost is high.

All inter-city and inter- IQSA RR transfers should be done by dedicated transfer vehicles. The system was very close to reaching this goal when multi-patient transfer vehicles were put into operation. This occurred in Sudbury, the same place where they built a "holding room" for patients at the airport. Flights were often delayed because ambulances were taking too long to arrive and transfer the patient off or on the plane. The holding room, or in transport terms a "terminal," allowed patient and escort to wait in comfort for an ambulance while the plane was free to continue with the next patient. Some may ask why it took so long for an ambulance to arrive. Generally, it was the result of high call volume and not enough resources. Ambulances were often diverted to higher priority calls. The stumbling blocks can now be overcome with a system designed for the province. The non-emergency inter-city and inter-IQSA RR scheduled bus transfer system would be the equivalent to the FedEx inter-city tractor trailer, used for long distances (under 500 km) and where speed is not a requirement. The patient transport buses will be on a schedule and will load and discharge patients only at terminals. Transportation to or from the terminal will be provided by a smaller van-type vehicle and may be managed by the municipality or a private service. Finally, the multi-patient transfer system can be brought back with confidence that its problems can be overcome.

The new transfer buses will be highway coach-type vehicles (similar to a Greyhound bus). These buses are designed with a lift to load four to six stretcher patients with reclining seating for another four to six patients but would be adaptable switching one setup for another. Every bus would be washroom equipped with storage for medical equipment, monitors, and oxygen onboard every bus. Staff will include the driver and one paramedic or nurse. Others that may be onboard include medical staff and escorts accompanying patients. Light lunches will be served on long-distance routes. The bus will be designed with a lift to enable easy loading of stretcher patients.

The main factor that will make the bus system a success where other attempts have failed is the terminal system and adhering to a schedule. Patients and their escort will not be picked up or let off at a tertiary hospital or a Focused Centre of Excellence by a bus unless the terminal is located there. But this is not recommended as the patient was rarely ready and often paramedics had to go to the patient's room resulting in long delays. Patients will be brought to the terminals by small-vehicle transfer services, or by local ambulance, to transfer onto or off a bus. Terminals for the large bus highway cruisers are usually located near the main gateways to a city and whenever possible, they will be at the same site as a primary care centre or primary emergency care centre. It is only at a terminal that patients are transferred onto or off the buses. Some may be going home, some may be going to tertiary care centres, and some may be going to or returning from Focused Centres of Excellence.

The bus transfer system proposed here assures that a schedule will be adhered to. Patients must be at the terminal holding room at the designated time or they will miss the connection. While at the terminal holding room the patient will be moved onto or off a special stretcher designed for the bus. Those being let off are able to wait in comfort until a short-haul transfer vehicle (i.e., smaller ambulance-type vehicle) or the inter- city bus arrives to pick them up or in some cases the inter-regional bus.

FedEx decides on the correct mode of transportation depending on distance, volume, and time required and the cost. If time is not a significant factor, a tractor trailer may be used on long distances. But if time is limited, an airplane might be used. If the distances are very long, they might use only airplanes. The IQSA health care transport system and FedEx's would be very similar in many ways. Both the IQSA health care system and FedEx use planes for long distances. Both systems use small vehicles for door-to-door delivery with the health care system using EMS ambulances or ambulance-type private vehicles (with no emergency lights). The primary difference is inter-city where FedEx often uses tractor trailers rather than planes because it is more economical; but this would also depend on other factors such as the state of infrastructure and traffic volume. Factors such as these will help FedEx decide whether land or air is the best choice.

The health care system has no equivalent to FedEx's tractor trailers. This may be because the use of tractor trailers requires terminals for offloading, sorting, and transferring to smaller vehicles for door-to-door delivery. If buses were used, they too would require a terminal where the patients would be transferred to other vehicles for the next leg of their trip. The government has been reluctant to do this because of the added expense. They may believe that the demand for the service may not be high enough to warrant the investment, but this would not be the case with the

IQSA system. This method is not only more practical and efficient it also has the added benefit of placing less demand on local ambulance services so that they are better able to respond to emergencies. The bus system will closely adhere to a schedule. Disembarking or loading, the bus will occur only at a terminal All will be strategically located. When possible being located at some E-Stat centres (combination centre) would be best because staff at these centres may be able at times to assist patients. All escorts and paperwork must be with the patient at the time of boarding.

The health system uses ambulances or similar vehicles for short haul door-to-door delivery. Because of this government has not seen a need for terminals. However, their absence results in many delays, requires smaller vehicles for long trips, increases the number of trips, and in cases where an ambulance is used, it takes them much farther out of their local coverage area thereby increasing the time it takes to put them back into emergency response mode.

When patients are not ready to transfer or the hospital is not ready for admission, delays result. What does this mean? For the IQSA system it means that as the volume of patients increases and more patients are required to travel farther, the use of scheduled bus service and terminals will prove their worth. The continued use of small vehicles without buses would require many more such vehicles, making it very uneconomical.

In Ontario, municipalities are tasked with providing 911 services including paramedic/ambulance services for their citizens. Municipalities do not want to provide services outside their boundaries where they do not collect taxes. Where private transfer services exist, the workload on municipal ambulance services will be reduced. But if the private service cannot keep up with the call volume, the local ambulance will be required to assist. In places where there is no private transfer service the ambulance will do all transfers. Many of these transfers cover long distances to other cities that may in the future be done by the bus system. All emergencies will continue to be done by ambulance.

The city transfer services will be responsible for patient transport to and from the terminal locally within the city. As an example, some patients would be picked up and taken to their home, hospital or clinic while others would be dropped off at the terminal to await the bus for an inter-city or inter-IQSA RR transfer. The buses only travel between terminals. Patients travelling more than five hours between destinations should fly.

Some beds currently in the health care system will be tertiary care beds. Patients that require these beds will be coming from Focused Centres of Excellence. Sometimes while at the tertiary hospital a patient will require a test such as a CT or MRI scan as ordered by the focused specialist overseeing their care. The smallest tertiary hospitals do not have this equipment. As in the past, many of these hospitals are just too small to warrant the large investment required for such equipment. The need for specialized equipment (MRI, CT, PET, etc.) for a patient at a tertiary care hospital or any other facility in the IQSA system could result in a temporary transfer to IQSA RR regional hospital or a local Focused Centre of Excellence whichever has the equipment and is closer. (which in many cases will be the same) to have the test done. The patient will be returned afterward. Finding a new way to share the equipment among many of these tertiary hospitals could be done by placing the required equipment on trucks and have a scheduled rotation that includes all required sites. Depending on demand, the medical equipment truck may be shared among more than one IQSA RR. This is a very old solution that was done in California in the 1970s.

We think of transportation in the health care field in very limited terms. Yes, transporting patients is a major portion of the work, but what we also need to start doing is investigating the transport of equipment. Ct, MRI, PET scanners, and radiation therapy machines, just to name a few. A bunker type garage would accommodate trucks that transport equipment that produce radiation so that only the patient is exposed. The specialist required for the use of the equipment would oversee the use of the equipment remotely. Transportation of patients is still the priority as we move through the transformation of the health care system, but other needs might be considered along the way.

Chapter Highlights

Currently, non-emergency transportation of patients is done by the public ambulance service (Emergency Medical Services) and private services where they exist. They use small vehicles and transport one patient at a time which is a very inefficient way to move patients. To meet the needs of the IQSA system, the transport business will need to be updated with a scheduled bus service. The system presented here will work well for a long time to come.

CHAPTER 11

IQSA Health Care Facilities

One of the greatest challenges facing the current system of health care is alternate level of care (ALC) patients. These are patients that no longer require hospital care but can not manage on their own and are waiting for a nursing home bed. Ontario has a chronic shortage of nursing home beds and this has resulted in many hospital beds being occupied for a longer duration than need be. In Sudbury, at times this has nearly reached up to one quarter of the total beds available in the local hospital.

It is imperative to find solutions for this problem. Ontario has announced that it will be building more nursing home beds which will help, but they will not be building enough to solve the problem or keep up with demand. Only a new approach will realize the answers we need.

Let's look at the types of continuing care that we do have:

Home care: government funded, income based, for those that live in their own home but need assistance. They must be mobile on their own, able to take their own medications without assistance, able to prepare some of their own meals, and are able to feed themselves or have other family members able to assist. Being able to do their own housekeeping is a plus but home care can assist.

Retirement homes: accommodation is privately funded. A nurse is on duty at all times. Some additional care may be government funded with specialized health professionals making visits. Seniors must be mobile on their own and able to take their own medication. Housekeeping is provided along with meals, and laundry services are available. A health care provider is in the building at all times. In the IQSA system, those living in these homes are entitled to the same amount of time for care as those living in their own homes. Since housekeeping and meals are provided, most requests will be for personal care. The retirement home may have rules that restrict who they allow in. In most cases the person must be able to walk unassisted, is able to feed themselves, and is able to take their own prescription drugs. Some services are provided such as laundry at additional cost.

Nursing homes: government funded, income-based admission. Nursing homes and home care are the oldest established systems for those requiring care other than hospitals. If around the clock care or supervision is required, then nursing home care is the choice. Nursing homes provide meals, laundry housekeeping, bathing, personal care, medication dispensing, feeding, and will accept patients that require mobility assistance. All required care is provided. Many are considered a public facility and so the government will subsidize costs for those unable to afford the care.

Hospice care: this may be partially government funded or private run non-profit with donation-funded short-term care for those that are suffering a terminal illness. All care is provided 24/7 along with all other services required for the duration.

Group homes: these homes are for those that are mentally or physically disabled but are not necessarily considered senior. These homes provide 24/7 care in all the same areas of care similar to nursing homes. They are subsidized by the government.

Focused Living: this is a newly proposed continuing care classification to alleviate problems concerning alternate level of care patients. Accommodation would be privately funded but rent controls would limit rent increases. Only nursing care and house keeping would be government funded, similar to home care. Focused living accommodation can be found for patients but it all depends on the amount and type of care required. The government will not be able to build enough nursing home facilities for all that require assistance but maybe if the problem was approached in a new way, it may be possible to provide care for many that do not need 24/7 care. What is required is not new specialized accommodation so much as care, and so this area is where efforts should be concentrated.

The focused living plan calls for working with some landlords of rental properties to designate their buildings or a portion of their buildings (i.e., adjoining floors of a high-rise) to what is known in the IQSA Health Care System as "Focused Living." As an example, to qualify a landlord would apply to have their building or a cluster of apartments designated as "focused living." To meet some client's needs, a few renovations would be required in some of the units. The standard bathtub will be changed to a walk-in tub or a shower with room to sit. Clients of focused living must be able to walk without assistance and able to feed themselves. Assistance with bathing, clothing, light housekeeping, and some food preparation will be provided if required. Rent of apartments is not subsidized, only the care provided is paid by the taxpayer as it would if the client were "home care". Those requiring more care than is available with home care, but not 24/7 care, may be suitable for Focused Living accommodation.

Those that cannot afford to rent an entire apartment or prefer not to, will still be allowed to move in but will be provided with one room in one of the apartments. Rental of the room would be less than for the whole apartment. plus, more people could be accommodated in the other rooms.

By creating Focused Living, it will allow personal support workers (PSWs) and others that provide care to do so with greater ease and efficiency. With patients being closer together there is less travel time and PSWs will have more time and are able to visit more patients rather than being on the road.

Focused Living accommodation in the IQSA system requires a shift to put the emphasis on providing care, the type of care and the amount of care. It is not bricks and mortar that is needed with this shift, so much as the care. Looking at it from this perspective opens the door to solving a long-standing problem.

The care time frames noted below in the continuing care guideline could assist in determining the proper accommodation for those requiring care. With these designations, choosing one will come down to the amount of care required:

1. Home care seniors: require care no more than one hour per day, two days per week.

2. Retirement homes: require care no more than two hours per day two days per week.

3. Focused Living: require care no more than two hours a day three days per week. (Time may increase)

4. Nursing home: require care 24 hours a day seven days a week.

5. Hospice care: short term care 24 hours a day seven days a week.

6. Group home: long-term care for those with mental or physical disabilities and may require 24 hours a day seven days a week care

Some of those in nursing homes may qualify for "Focused Living." This may free up more beds at nursing homes for those requiring 24/7 care. In addition, more people will be accommodated sooner with Focused

Living in the IQSA system because the accommodation in many cases has already been built. It is truly about the care and not the bricks and mortar.

The fundamental change in health care described in this book will require a fiscal investment in some aspects of care, but because the hospitals already exist, much of that additional investment is contained. One-time funding for training will be required to upgrade the knowledge and skill level of some health care providers.

In addition to such funding, the following is a list of the facilities that comprise the IQSA Health Care System, some of which will also need capital to establish, but the amount may be reduced because of the change to larger facilities where sharing of staff and equipment will help. There are seven main types of facilities in the IQSA health care system. They are:

1. The nurse practitioner-led primary care clinics (note: some have already been built).

2. The paramedic-led primary emergency care centres (construction required).

3. The Focused Centres of Excellence staffed by specialists 24/7/365 (utilizing current hospital space).

4. The tertiary care hospitals (already in existence).

5. The hospital emergency departments (already in existence).

6. The health consultation centre (H2C) and the health transport centre (HTC) (construction required).

7. Medical transport terminals with holding rooms to be built in conjunction with #2 above, when possible (Construction required).

Note: An E-Stat centre is a site with a combination of services; the site will include primary emergency care staffed by paramedics along with an ambulance base. Options are a primary care site staffed by nurse practitioners. Many other optional services may be included at the E-Stat that will be determined by the municipalities and the province.

Listed below are some additional factors to be considered regarding facilities:

1. All primary care will slowly shift to the nurse practitioner-led clinics. Some have already been built but many more will need to be constructed, although not as many as one might think. Most of these clinics will be in operation 24/7, replacing many physician offices with their limited hours. This will mean that fewer clinics can serve more people. Included in the change will be a shift to telemedicine. Patients with minor aliments will be able to video conference with their nurse practitioner at the clinic at appointed times, and receive prescriptions electronically sent to the drug store of their choice (which was often done during Covid). This will also reduce the number of patients coming to the clinic.

2. The next fundamental change needed to build the IQSA health care system involves the construction of paramedic-led primary emergency care centres. Where possible, the primary emergency care centres will be built adjacent to an ambulance service base (EMS) in what is called an E-Stat centre.

3. The Focused Centres of Excellence provide care to all patients that require admission and are a major part of the IQSA Health Care System. They are distributed equally among all IQSA RRs and are managed by the hospital board where they are located. The Focused Centres of Excellence will use beds currently in the system as designated by the province and IQSA RR in consultation.

4. The tertiary care hospitals will provide extended care for those requiring it after discharge from a Focused Centre of Excellence. All beds not used for Focused Centres of Excellence will be designated as tertiary care beds. Tertiary care will be managed by the same board that manages the hospital currently. Some hospitals will be a combination tertiary care site, Focused Centre of Excellence site, and emergency department site, but not all. Relatively few hospitals will have Focused Centre of Excellence units.

5. All those hospitals that currently have an emergency department will continue to operate them in the same way.

6. The health consultation centre (H2C) will be a new entity and will provide service to the whole province. Funding is required but because the physicians there are already employed in the system, it should only require an outlay for the facility. The H2C's main objective is to provide a second opinion on the treatment for all patients, and to coordinate their care through the system.

If we go back in time, it may be possible to pinpoint some of the changes that have contributed to overcrowding in hospital emergency departments. Today's family physician no longer does house calls or time-consuming procedures in the office, such as placing a cast on a fractured limb or suturing a laceration. This work has been passed on to the emergency department because lengthy procedures cut back on the time a physician has to see additional patients at the office and this costs him time and money. Some patients go to the emergency department because doctors' offices or walk-in clinics are not open 24/7. These problems result in patients going to the only facility that is open, the emergency department. The whole system needs to be open when required by the patient.

The change to an all-specialist system will result in fewer if any family physicians providing primary care. New ways of providing this vital service need to be found. If primary care is divided into office-type primary care and primary emergency care, the two professions best prepared to fill in for a family physician would be the registered nurse practitioner (RNP) and paramedic professions. By doing this it will be possible to shift some work currently done in the hospital emergency department back to "out-of-hospital" care as it once was. The primary care change has started with the creation of nurse practitioner clinics. This was a great first step that can be expanded on because it has proven its worth. Now the system can take another step and create primary emergency care centres with paramedics.

All main components of the IQSA system will function 24/7. This will result in better utilization of facilities and equipment and with fewer facilities and less equipment being required. As an example, it will no longer be necessary to have three scanners working eight hours a day each when one scanner will work 24 hours a day. It will no longer be necessary to have thousands of physicians each with their own office when one facility can accommodate many physicians and offices can be used and shared as necessity dictates. In addition, staffing requirements may be reduced depending on the staffing configuration (e.g., eight-hour vs twelve-hour shifts).

Nurse practitioners have already opened nurse practitioner-led clinics that have proven to be quite effective. However, paramedics have yet to open primary emergency care centres. Paramedics are the best choice for these centres. With their education and experience in emergency care it would take little additional training to prepare them for work at a primary emergency care centre. Eventually, a university degree program could be introduced for a paramedic practitioner program.

All primary emergency centres will post all treatable conditions at the entrance and online. If the patient feels that they have a condition that is treatable at the primary emergency care centre, the patient will first call

Telehealth and receive an access number. Telehealth will direct the patient to the appropriate facility. This will also apply to primary care. Telehealth is a telephone service in Ontario where nurses provide medical advice or directs patients to the appropriate care provider. In this case, the Telehealth nurse will obtain all required information and forward it to the appropriate centre.

All primary emergency care provided by paramedics is through medical directives and protocols that are evidence based. This may only change if a specialist has been contacted. Care may include issues related to asthmatics, diabetics, epileptics, and minor lacerations requiring dressings, suturing, casting fractures of limbs prior to transfer to a focused centre for orthopedics, minor concussions, minor ear and eye infections, diarrhea, constipation, back pain, and vertigo or other conditions as care evolves. Care for some of these conditions can be provided with current paramedic training levels but some conditions will require additional training.

Paramedics are just shy of where they need to be regarding education, to provide all "out-of-hospital" primary emergency care. The centres could open now with the current level of training being an advanced-care paramedic with five years experience, but the shift to providing care for all urgent patients not requiring admission would not be complete. This benchmark would be important in bringing true "timely" primary emergency care to all communities, large and small. In addition, the hospital emergency department would only receive meaningful overload relief by reaching this benchmark.

During the transition to nurse practitioner clinics, modifications in training were made allowing nurse practitioners to prescribe medication and, in the beginning, did not include narcotics. The transition for paramedics would require some additional training in suturing, imaging fractures with ultrasound or assisting with remote X-ray imaging, setting fractured long bones in a cast before referral to a specialist, and operating a mini-laboratory for some types of blood tests. A few of these skills have been done by paramedics in some jurisdictions.

An E-Stat centre is a facility with a combination of services. It might be a primary care site as well as a primary emergency care site and may include an ambulance station or a medical transport terminal for buses. Just as a house or any building must meet construction standards, it is suggested that E-Stat centres meet provincial regulations in staffing, design, function, and hours of operation. This may assure that all E-Stat centres are recognized by the public and they will know what to expect as far as services provided, time of operation, and type of staffing. A somewhat similar look would assist the public with identification and all would function the same for the care provided. This would lessen public confusion in trying to understand the types of care or service provided, or how it is accomplished (the process), and lessen orientation time for staff, plus lower capital costs and standardize staffing levels. Cancer care Ontario is an example of a provider that has set up branches in strategic locations and has done much to standardize treatment.

A capital investment in paramedic-led primary emergency care facilities province-wide will do more than just improve 24/7 access to primary emergency care and decrease the load on the hospital emergency department. It will reserve the time emergency physicians have for those patients that are most in need of their expertise, expertise that only they can provide. Those municipalities that choose to add additional services and create an E-Stat centre may find that they will help reduce the cost of providing those additional services through reductions in real estate and utility costs and supplies, plus it may promote new ways of collaborating.

The past decade or so has seen a change with the province and municipalities assisting with some of these costs for those physicians in family health teams. If primary emergency care centres or nurse practitioner clinics were widespread, the province, municipality or both would need to invest in the infrastructure just as was done with the family health teams. Building the centres as part of the IQSA system would mean saving on some of these office costs that individual physicians had. As a municipal public facility, they would also be non-profit facilities. Rent fees would not be required and property taxes might be waved.

In the IQSA system, construction material and equipment would be purchased in bulk, resulting in savings. Utility costs should be lower as more services share the facility and we build them to the latest insulation and efficiency standards. The Ontario Ministry of Health and Long-Term Care realized just how much bulk-purchase savings can amount to when they bulk-purchased CT scanners for Ontario hospitals and saved million over their original estimates.

Many areas of health care have fallen out of synchronization with the way our society lives. It has been trending toward slower service and higher costs. Frankly, health care no longer matches our modern "first world" high standard of living expectations. These trends can be reversed when we move to the IQSA system. E-Stat centres, if developed, may easily extend cooperation between public services. If this idea takes hold, Ontario will be much better prepared for emergencies. All services at the E- Stat will receive information concerning emergencies at the same time, possibly improving response and preparation time. Patients that come to E-Stat but are not primary emergency care patients, will be cared for by a nurse practitioner in their clinic if located there, unless they need to transfer the patient to an emergency department. Every E-Stat is linked to every other part of the health care system through the health consultation centre and may be able to divert some patients at times to less busy locations.

Chapter Highlights

The IQSA system introduces some new ways to provide services using primarily existing facilities. Some facilities may require new investment but most of the change revolves around existing facilities functioning in new more efficient ways that fit together into the new IQSA bigger picture. Reconfiguring existing facilities into the IQSA system is designed to provide the finest service when the patient requires it, day or night, for people living anywhere in the province, and this is accomplished through the health transport centre.

The primary emergency care centres may be stand-alone centres or they may be combined with other services at an E-Stat centre. The two main services provided might be the primary emergency care centre and an ambulance base. An optional service may include a nurse practitioner primary-care clinic. Some centres will also be the location of the inter-city or inter-IQSA RR transfer bus service terminal complete with a holding room for those on stretchers awaiting connections. Talks with local municipal and provincial representatives will determine which optional services, if any, will be located at the E-Stat centre if there are E-Stat centres.

CHAPTER 12

Health Care Safety
and Global Opportunity

Health Care Safety

Some of these ideas for health care safety that have been already discussed include checklists, using standard care evidence-based practices, video conferencing with a focused specialist, and a virtual consult specialist for a second opinion for all patients. More efforts must also be made to reduce errors. The IQSA system will use barcoding or QR technology for all patients in an effort to reduce errors. All patients admitted will receive a coded wristband from the start of admission that will remain with the patient for the entire length of stay. This will make the system safer for patients, reducing the chances of giving a drug or test to the wrong patient. All coded wrist bands will be scanned just before a patient receives medication or treatment.

Time is money and the health care system is expensive. When errors are made, it may not only cause harm to the patient, it slows the entire system down. Errors take time to correct. Time that could be spent treating a new patient is instead spent on treating the patient that suffered as a result of an error. The Ontario compensation board knows that the longer it takes to return the patient to a productive working life, the greater the cost. These delays are costly to the system in other ways because the longer it takes to treat a patient, the worse the condition often becomes, requiring extended treatment and thereby driving up costs. Reducing errors through a new system of checks and balances can be done.

Checklists included with standard care follow through step-by step for all procedures. This should act as reference material to reduce errors. Today's technology makes it much easier to reference material. Creating and referencing digital checklists are a common way to help eliminate errors. Airline pilots go through many checklists all designed to eliminate errors and increase safety. It is done through electronic means to prevent missing a step. This mindset needs to carry over to health care with all providers, including physicians and nurses, using this method.

Simulator technology is used in many industries but once again, the airline industry has been a leader. Some errors may be eliminated by having regulatory colleges demand that health care providers, including physicians, practice on simulators. Such technology, which is relatively new in the medical field compared to the airline industry, may well become much more prominent as it becomes clear that this is an easy way to keep skills honed and up to date.

Both manikin and desktop simulator programs could prove their usefulness, though to date, both have seen limited usage. Paramedics have been using manikins to assist with training for decades. The training manikins are used annually or more often and the practice is mandatory. The manikins have gradually advanced to the point where they are able to assist in training for many more conditions than in the past. In the case of physicians, it would currently be difficult to build manikins that would be complex enough to simulate all the work that they do. A surgeon, for example, may need a computer program simulator designed for their specialty. The monitor screen displays, the patient image, and various scenarios programmed into the computer are used to simulate the patient's condition. This practice should increase the safety factor.

The benefits of practice can not be ignored. The professional colleges responsible for each profession should provide annual mandatory practice sessions for all health care providers, including doctors and nurses. Online practice sessions would be able to accommodate more people at less cost and could be done annually, benefiting providers and the patient. Computer programs have advanced to the point where surgeons may be able to train online for some procedures, gaining valuable practice. Increasingly, surgery is becoming computer assisted with surgeons manipulating robotic arms while performing micro-surgery.

Simulator training is commonplace in other high-pressure high-skilled professions. Many airlines and their regulators require pilots to practice on simulators annually and when training to operate a new aircraft. The training is very intense. The more complex the job, the more it may include working with technology. In Ontario, paramedics have been practicing on simulators (manikins) for years. In the last few years, nurses have joined in and medical students are also beginning to see the benefits. These benefits should be carried over to all practicing physicians where once a year they are scenario tested.

A demanding job needs to be done safely. Going back to the airline industry example, pilots not only practice on simulators, they are also required to go through medical checkups on a regular basis to assure that they are fit to provide the service. All health care providers should be physically fit to assure that they can safely provide the service. The following is a recommendation in a report by Lisa Priest that indicates (paraphrased) we have higher medical checkup standards for airline pilots than for physicians and surgeons in Canada.... retesting should be standard for all physicians. [xxv] In Ontario, having a medical checkup is part of the paramedic's job requirements and is done in conjunction with their driver's license renewal which they must have. New regulations, if required, for physician and nurse employment may require medical checkups with a physical and psychological component.

In the past, both paramedics on board the ambulance were equally trained. This provided the benefit of someone being readily available to consult regarding diagnosis and treatment. Contact with a physician in emergency was possible but rarely exercised because emergency physicians are so busy so they had to rely on each other. Each paramedic had their own assigned duties but the duties were interchangeable between the two (i.e., driver or patient attendant) and were usually rotated daily. This safety approach was exponentially magnified with the amount of experience that each paramedic team member had. Many potential problems were avoided. This was a safety factor that was never officially recognized. Ontario has two types of paramedics working on ambulances, primary care paramedic and advanced-care paramedic. Having two advanced-care paramedics work together was not considered necessary. It was decided that better utilization of the ACP would occur if they were spread out and teamed up with primary care paramedics (PCP). In the IQSA Health Care System, to reduce the chance of errors, the focused specialist and the consult specialist will have the same qualifications.

Some will say that IQSA is just too expensive, that we cannot afford it. I don't agree but then I say if the health care portion of the budget pie is too small, let's bake a larger pie. Global opportunities are out there. Health care does not have to be such a drain on the public purse. The system could be an income generator in its own right. For-profit endeavours by public health care will be encouraged. Profit from these ventures will go back into the system to offset implementation costs and lower operating costs. Many areas of the IQSA Health Care System are designed for safety as has been explained in previous chapters, but they also serve as part of a process that will provide faster and lower-cost quality service.

The health care system is costly and becoming more so as time goes on. This was noted in a study by the OECD in which I paraphrase, three quarters of health spending is provided by the taxpayer and all OECD countries in the last 20 years have health spending rising faster than economic growth.[xxvi] To help sustain it we should look at ways to lessen the cost to the taxpayer.

Striving to meet Ontario's health care needs and those of all Canadians is a great goal. But to achieve excellence, and sustainability, may require more funding than is foreseeably available through Canadian government sources. To overcome this, we should look at what other industries do. In business, truly successful endeavours in our modern age migrate from a purely local or domestic focus to include a global focus. In this case I am referring to what is commonly called medical tourism. Canadians should not shy away from this, especially in areas in which we are strong. Health care is one of those areas and is also a major economic driver.

It may also help stem the tide of Canadians that travel abroad for health care. Jane Stevenson reports on Statistics Canada, I paraphrase in 2019, 217,500 fellow Canadians went outside the country to get care.[xxvii] Our economy is growing faster in the services sector than in many other areas. As the economy grows, it benefits all Canadians. Health care is becoming a prime concern and one of the largest growth areas for many countries as their populations age. This includes our own population.

Many of the clinics that care for medical tourists do so with leading-edge treatments or equipment that may not be available in the patient's own country. Additional public income may be used for the purchase of equipment if we don't already have it. Altogether, Ontarians could increase the benefit to the public by approaching medical tourism in new and innovative ways. If we use the automobile as an example, it turns out that in the early days, cars were very expensive. So, few were produced, only the rich could afford to purchase them. What this also meant was that high profit margins were necessary for corporations because of limited production. A large portion of that cash flow was used to develop leading-edge technology. Things such as new and more powerful engines, better drive trains, long-wearing materials, and safer cars all around. As mass production took over, those innovations made their way into cars that the average worker could afford. Without the huge inflow of cash relative to production in the early stages, it would have taken much longer to create these advances.

Let's do for health care what was done for the automobile. How would medical tourism work in a public system? It can be done. Just as the Liquor Control Board of Ontario is public and generates profits for the public. Health care can do this also. Let me explain how it may work. Health care will remain a public entity for Ontarians but foreign medical tourists would be required to pay for services. Profits from the services would be reinvested in the public system to assist in meeting the health care needs of Ontarians and might also help spur innovation.

Medical Tourism Model

    – Medical tourism is only allowed if Ontarians can receive care at a Focused Centre of Excellence within three weeks. Only then will specialists be able to do medical tourism work. Medical tourist patients will not go to the front of the line but will be scheduled in the same way as all other patients.

    – All work is done at public Focused Centres of Excellence.

    – All specialists will be required to work in the public system but will have the option to participate in the medical tourism program.

    – All medical tourists will be billed by the public administration on behalf of the specialist taking the following into consideration.

      a. The public administration (PA) of the Focused Centre of Excellence will calculate the fee to cover the cost of wages of public staff employed for medical tourist care and the cost of equipment on a shared time basis, plus any other supplies, and add it to the bill.

b. The PA will charge a fee for rent of public space for the treatment and recovery of the tourist at the focused unit.

c. The PA will charge a fee for administration (i.e., billing).

d. The PA will estimate the cost of utilities and any other overhead costs and add it to the bill.

*All of the above is calculated at cost and then a 25% markup is applied for public system profit. The focused specialist's fee is added to the bill. Each specialist will decide their own fee. The cost estimate of the work will be provided to the medical tourist before work is done and full payment in advance will be required.

As long as Ontarians receive care within three weeks at the Focused Centre of Excellence, all specialists at the site will have the option of earning extra income above what others earn in the public system. In other words, they will earn a public wage and a private wage if they participate in the medical tourism program.

The morale of all health care providers will improve as they raise their standard of knowledge and practice and are able to help more people get the care they require in a timely fashion. With IQSA, volume, specialization, and new processes will lower the per capita cost of care, it will save more lives with 24/7 care specialists onsite at all times in all categories of care, and it will generate income for the system to help offset costs and provide incentives for health care providers.

Another benefit of the medical tourist program is that Canadians will begin to get a true handle on the cost of health care. People will see and understand health care costs by reviewing the posted billing costs for medical tourism. Most Canadians do not understand what it costs to provide the health care they receive, and most administrations do not see the full picture or where efficiencies could be made. More information is needed, and this program will provide it, adding income that will be used to keep us ahead of the ever-rising health care cost curve.

Some may criticize the IQSA system as not being affordable. This is not true. It's the current system which is well on its way to not being affordable as it continuously demands more funding to operate in the old way. Governments have compensated by reducing staffing and closing hospital beds or entire hospitals. This does not mean the current system will disappear. The road we are on will continue to witness falling access and rising costs with fewer and fewer Ontarians gaining access in a timely fashion. In other words, health care is becoming exclusive, just as the fine old cars of days gone by. They too, like health care today, provided quality work and fine service–but only for a few. The few fortunate to gain access. This needs to change.

Until now there's been no viable alternative. Now with the optional IQSA system, our current health care system will no longer be required to work with a smaller piece of a shrinking pie. With this new system, the answer is to bake a larger pie. In other words, invite patients from around the globe here, to Canada, to receive some of the best care available anywhere. The difference being that they would have to pay for their care out-of-pocket.

Other provinces may see the benefit of delegating out some of their health care requirements to a jurisdiction that can provide excellent care faster, and may have their health care insurance plans pay to send some of their patients to the IQSA system in Ontario. This agreement would be in keeping with the Canada Health Act and could be an agreement between provinces, paid for with public funds. The one primary consideration for other provinces to participate would be a commitment to sending a specific number of patients for care under a long-term contract in the area of 30 years or more.

People in countries outside of Canada may also want to take advantage of the excellent care at reasonable cost and may have the cash or insurance that will pay for it. Changing to the IQSA system will require an infusion of cash, but the IQSA time frame will lessen the impact and the payback in savings will be realized in proportion to implementation. If the funding to transition to the IQSA system is in short supply, then let's look for additional funds elsewhere. Medical tourism may be the answer. All Focused Centres of Excellence will allow specialists working there to take on additional work to increase their income, and in turn, increase public self-funding. Other government services such as the post office and the LCBO raise money for government coffers. Health care can also.

How might this work? Specialists that want to take advantage of the medical tourism program would apply to the public administration managing the Focused Centre of Excellence. The IQSA system recommends that this administration be the hospital board. The hospital board would decide if private care may be provided at one of their Focused Centres of Excellence based on the criteria that follows:

1. If the focused centre is able to meet the maximum wait of no more than three weeks for care for Ontarians.

2. The need for such a service must be demonstrated or be able to be generated. This means that through advertising and anticipated demand assessments or other methods, it could be determined that enough medical tourists could be enticed to come here so that the program would be a success.

3. The service can create a profit to be applied to public care.

4. Separate financial books would be kept for medical tourism.

5. Separate performance indicators would be kept.

Because public facilities and staff would be used, the specialist would not need to invest huge sums of money to set up their own clinic or sustain the high overhead costs of running their own facility. It is a ready-made system. In return for using public property and employees, the income generated by bringing in foreign patients would be divided. The cost to the public system would be reimbursed along with a return on investment, and the specialist working privately would decide their fee. The billing invoice would combine the two and the public facility would bill the medical tourist patient. Competition on setting physician fees would be allowed. Foreign medical tourists would not receive priority but would need to wait up to the maximum of three weeks as Ontarians would. If Ontarians are found to be waiting longer than three weeks for care, then the medical tourist program would be suspended until such time as the maximum three-week wait was regained.

As one Focused Centre of Excellence generates income from the program, it will be divided between the public and the specialist. There may be many places to invest the public portion, such as to assist in introducing another Focused Centre of Excellence or to bring in new equipment and the latest treatment regimen. Working in the global health care market will have us striving to remain at the forefront with the latest innovations. Regardless of whether funding from this source is needed, the system needs to take the leap to become a global health care service sector leader. Many countries are already well on their way and Canada will soon be left far behind if we do not take hold of this opportunity. Some Canadians already go elsewhere for their medical care. This is not a good sign. It may be because of the long wait times but in some cases, the treatment here is not cutting edge.

Advancing the system by using our expertise to help people with health care needs worldwide is the way to go. This is similar to many other businesses that supply local populations but still sell their goods and services worldwide. In fact, for many private businesses, restricting sales locally would make them economically non-viable. This would apply to automobile and airplane makers, furniture and appliance manufacturers, clothing companies, and on a national scale, grocery stores and possibly some chain restaurants that purchase food in bulk for hundreds of restaurants.

The differences in cost per capita of health care in different provinces is large but not attributed to scale. The current health care system does not create an environment which would allow the system to benefit much from economies of scale in a meaningful way. The following report taken from the Canadian Press article in which the analysis of health care spending by Toronto based Dale Orr Economic Insight indicates (paraphrased) greater population, demographic differences and economies of scale would not account for the high-cost differences.[xxviii]This statement refers to the per capita differences in health care costs between provinces that they believe would not be accounted for by economies of scale among other factors. If we want economies of scale, the system must be designed to produce this outcome, otherwise it will not happen. The IQSA system can do this and in addition create equal access, plus will even out the large per capita cost differences between provinces. Although the following is in regards to negotiations between the federal government and a province, but the same could be said for talks between provinces as indicated by Katherine Fierlbeck where she highlights the following. (paraphrased) It shows us that caution is required when jurisdiction is shared, communication may improve, but it may also increase accountability problems. Predictability and stability are needed but so is accountability and transparency.[xxix]Unfortunately, the road to public health care economies of scale is clouded by decades of resistance.

Maybe before starting on the global medical tourism theme, we should first try at building the economies of scale at home. In these cases, such provinces would maintain their current hospitals as tertiary care hospitals but consider transferring some of the patients they have in the present system, that are not receiving care in a timely way, out-of-province to Focused Centres of Excellence. A maximum four days at an IQSA Focused Centre of Excellence should provide the time required to quickly set the patient on a course to the best recovery possible. Then the patient would return home or possibly to a tertiary hospital in the home area. This service would be faster, less costly, and of higher quality than in a smaller jurisdiction trying to provide every type of service required in small quantities, with possibly less experienced and less specialized staff.

Another option might be, rather than sending patients to the IQSA system in Ontario, other provinces could create their own IQSA system. But because other provinces are so much smaller than Ontario they would need to join with other provinces (e.g., Atlantic provinces or Prairie provinces forming a group) to increase patient numbers. The 23 categories of care that the IQSA Focused Centres of Excellence provide would be divided up between the participating provinces with each province specializing in the areas that they feel they would be best at providing. The IQSA system will maintain provincial control over health care budgets but will give them an option to join forces with other provinces to create the economies of scale plus enjoy benefits that they are not able to generate on their own. This does not mean the end of their local health care system. In fact, it will make it stronger because it will not be pulled in so many directions trying to provide all types of care. As in Ontario, beds not used for Focused Centres of Excellence would be used as tertiary care beds.

Ontario will benefit from the much shorter wait time for admission and IQSA can benefit other provinces in this way also. Bulk purchasing of medical supplies and drugs will also help lower costs and all will maintain their current health care system but specialize in new ways. Depending on the arrangement made between the provinces and the number of patients other provinces send to IQSA, the beds designated for tertiary care may increase.

For the Ontario IQSA system it has been suggested that if foreign patients can come here to Ontario for care, why not other Canadians. This may be an untapped market. So long as no one on the Ontario waiting list is waiting longer than three weeks for care, anyone, including other Canadians, should be able to receive care in Ontario and have the bill go to their provincial health insurance plan. Of course, this does not mean they go to the front of the line. They will be placed on the same list as all others in Ontario.

Most manufactured goods are produced in volume and stores like Walmart sell in volume. It is the modern standard in retail. Business grows in size because it is the most effective way to meet their own needs. Businesses that don't grow have a limited life span. Health care needs to move from the general hospital with the small "mom-and-pop" unit approach. It needs to surpass the regional approach and move to the specialized IQSA system. We can set a new standard by adopting a more modern business approach to the system. And this includes treating patients from across the country and around the world.

Ontario has the population to accomplish IQSA, but some medical or surgical conditions will exist where Ontario may not have sufficient volumes to maintain 24/7 service. It would be preferable, then, if Canadians from other provinces came here for care. However, if this could not be worked out, there are enough people in other parts of the world that would love to come to Canada for our health care.

Letting the world know Ontario's IQSA Health Care System is open for global business can help them and will in turn help us. Selling raw materials and commodities to the world is what Canadians are good at and known for but soon the future will include many additional services. With the IQSA system, health care will be one of them. We are all shareholders in the business of public health care and any change must be to the benefit of the Ontario public. The IQSA system is designed to do this. And one way to assist the transition is to do what is counter intuitive and open up health care to serve the many, either within Canada or globally.

Any time Ontarians have a product or service that can benefit the world and generate income, especially for public services, we should not sit on it. All Ontarians should take full advantage of their knowledge, skills, and resources in the global economy and that includes those in health care. Patients will come here for the best health care possible, but these people need to know that Ontario would welcome them. **Just bring your credit card.**

Health care medical tourism will place us on the map in a big way and lower the tax burden. Package deals that include air, focused accommodation, and care (all inclusive) will draw large numbers of patients. Packages could also include tertiary care at a hotel with private nurses if required. People will give up their trips to their favourite vacation destinations (i.e., Caribbean, Europe) for the best care available. If we need to look elsewhere to bump up volume and make the system economically viable, then this is what could be done. Canadians might support this provided their needs were met.

Canada has the expertise that the world needs and wants. We can provide that opportunity here but the current system makes it increasingly difficult. Canadians are among the best educated and trained people in the world. Our expertise in medicine, which is well-known, will become world renowned. From research to our leading-edge tele-robotic surgery to our upcoming vaccine production, Canada has some of the best physicians, researchers, and hospitals in the world. Ontarians should capitalize on this growing industry. Our health care system could be a great source of income and when used to subsidize the cost of health care for Ontarians, it will help sustain the system. Medical tourism could be the next big economic driving force in Ontario. It should be explored.

Bringing in customers from abroad has been occurring for a long time. Post-secondary education can provide an example. Universities and colleges actively recruit foreign students, and some go beyond this by setting up campuses in foreign countries. These students actually add to the bottom line, enabling institutions to keep their heads above water. Canada has a reputation for quality education, and schools are taking advantage of this to help offset costs. It helps schools as well as the taxpayer. Health care is no different. Costs can be offset just as other public institutions have done. In so doing, other benefits will be realized. The current health system brings in patients from abroad on a humanitarian basis. More can be done.

Another stream of revenue that should be explored comes through public entrepreneurs. Often as an employee of the service they see opportunities for the public service to increase revenue. A reward for these ideas if implemented should be offered. This would be much like what private entrepreneurs do for private services. As such, they should be identified in the new IQSA system. Public entrepreneurs are not totally new to public services and have saved services millions or generated additional money for public services in a wide variety of ways. Public entrepreneurs do this through new and innovative ways that do not in any way diminish the current service, but only serve to improve it. This should be encouraged. By helping to offset public cost they should receive some monetary compensation as encouragement to them and any others with ideas. In Toronto, some large hospitals had very large empty lobbies (foyers) that they put to good use as revenue streams. One opened a food court and rented out space to fast food franchises and also opened a smaller version of a well-know drug store chain. Some decided to go into the lottery business and do good with 50/50 draws or other types of ticket sales.

The LCBO (Liquor Control Board of Ontario) is another example. It is a government-run enterprise that makes huge profits for Ontario. Hydro Quebec produces profits for its government by selling power to the US

and the Ontario Lottery and Gaming Corporation (OLG) is very successful at turning over huge profits to the government as well. Many public
sectors are feeling the pinch these days as governments tighten their belts,
but services such as these are not sitting back and are continuing to funnel
money into the system. They should be encouraged. Maybe in the future
health care can be added. Many corporations already see huge returns in
the health care sector, from pharmaceuticals to biotechnology. The question is: why not the public health care system?

The province of Ontario already spends 47% of its budget on health
care. Increases in the health budget cannot be expected to continue. Work
should seriously begin on finding ways to reduce the burden and one way
of doing this is not by reducing service, but expanding it through medical
tourism either nation wide or globally. Generating profits from this business venture will help offset the cost of health care to Ontarians.

In Deli, India, there is a company that has a modern office building filled with radiologists. They sit at their computer monitors reading
X-rays and other scans much as they do here, except the customers they
have are located worldwide. They are generating cash with their knowledge
and service. They guarantee a quick turnaround of 30 minutes or less. The
work that these radiologists do is possible because of the explosion in the
number of images that need reading and the fact that most images today
are digital. Where once there were three or four X-ray images per patient
to read, nowadays one scan may produce 600 images per patient. This
takes a lot of reading time. If there were more radiologists in Canada going
global like in India, the health care system could benefit from the injection
of additional cash. Letting possible income sit on the sidelines when it is
badly needed for the system is not forward thinking.

A problem that may arise is that as income is generated, many will
apply pressure to transfer that income into large salary increases that may
cancel out the gains for the public system. Hopefully allowing physicians or

others the right to earn extra income from medical tourism will help slow demands for higher salaries in the public sector. Another example might be governments that take that extra income into their coffers and use it in other places rather than health care. It would not be recommended.

Ontario's population is around 14 million. Building one system to manage the health care workload is possible. It is already under one public-payer system. The IQSA Health Care System is a large manageable system that is Integrated, Quality, Sustainable, Accessible and will transform health care.

Chapter Highlights

Canadians do not want to be second-class citizens to those that can afford to pay for care. Inviting paying patients here from other parts of the globe will benefit the system but they must not be given priority. It will also enable those physicians that want to earn additional income the opportunity to do so. By providing faster service to the Ontario public, they may provide a win-win situation for both the Canadian public and them. It is human nature for some to be very competitive. Given this opportunity many may excel in their field adding to those already considered leading world experts. This should not be discouraged. IQSA Health Care System can greatly benefit from medical tourism and other forms of income generation which, to a degree, is already happening. But more can be done. Canadians might support these ideas because they want public care to continue.

CONCLUSION

In 2014, 30 countries across six continents with 65 global health leaders came together to discuss what makes a high-performing health care system. In its report from KPMG called *Staying Power*, the leaders stated that (paraphrased) the drive for improvement and innovation is necessary for success but must be accompanied with the ability to stay the course for real progress[xxx] The health care system is under government oversight and governments and policies can change every four years. The IQSA Health Care System can't be fully implemented in four years and therein lies the problem. Change that may be close to making a difference may be stopped or reversed before the full benefit is realized. This is what happened to the Local Health Integration Networks (LHIN).

Indeed, a fully Integrated, Quality, Sustainable, and Accessible health care system needs to be implemented, and we must stay the course with it and no longer try to fix our health care system willy-nilly. Yes, decision time has come. While much can be done through telemedicine, the IQSA system will require many to travel longer distances to see a specialist for care. Will Ontarian's insist on all care being close to home provided by those struggling to keep up? We will soon know. In an increasingly complex system, the pressure will continue to build thereby burning out more professionals until we realize that the health care system can be managed much better if it were divided into larger but less diverse sectors for each IQSA RR. Each Focused Centre of Excellence will have a concentrated focus on a smaller sector of the health care system and with a maximum of three types of care per IQSA RR, it will not overwhelm administration.

The general guide for the IQSA system should include the following goals. Outline the standard care protocols and medical directives process for standard care. Design the facilities to enable the process to be achieved. establish the time frame to provide the care. Train the staff to match the process and to work within the time frame. Locate the facilities in the best locations. Educate the public on the new system. Constantly review everything and update as required.

Maybe it's time for health care to take the next step. The current stress levels are leading to unhappy patients and depression among health care providers, including physicians. Patient adverse effects may increase if the system does not change. The problems can be corrected but the root of the problem must be recognized. It is not too late; we can get it together and make it work for everyone.

Large health care systems are in existence and one is Kaiser Permanente in the US. They are doing very well and are growing. Kaiser Permanente, a health care system based in California combines its own hospitals and clinics with a non-profit insurance plan. They made an announcement as reported by Abby Goodnough and I paraphrase, that they would open their own medical school in the state in 2019,[xxxi]. Kaiser Permanente is recognized as a leader in health care solutions, with 10 million patients covered under their insurance plan, 38 hospitals and 18,000 doctors **It is building toward the advantages that we already have but don't take advantage of.** They know larger is better and that small efficiencies on a large scale add up to big benefits. Ontario's public system includes a very large public health care insurance plan with 14.5 million patients insured, 146 hospitals and employs 31,500 doctors and trains them. This is our public system. Kaiser Permanente has achieved what Ontario currently has and will be moving on to the next step. Ontario's system is large but has not followed through with full integration. It will not remain the same forever. The two choices are, break it down into smaller units or go with the larger proposed IQSA system. Kaiser Permanente knows the advantages in being big and integrated and they may recognize the advantages to large scale specialization. I don't think that they will go in the opposite direction and create many more small units once they have read this book. In the mean time Ontario may go with small scale privatization losing our advantage. Costs will increase along with pressure for the public sector to shed more and more services. Our public system has had the Kaiser Permanente advantage for years with more benefits to come if the recommendations in this book are followed. All we have to do is take advantage of what we already have.

The IQSA system could begin having an impact in as little as two years with some new facilities being built or renovations to existing building might take a little less time. New staff could be trained in this same timeframe. Going private will also take at least this long. The private sector will need to build or renovate facilities also. With really good pay staff will leave the public sector for the private.

I wish we could turn back the clock to the days when your family doctor could take care of all your health needs and you could get an appointment with them the same day you needed it. I wish our local hospital could look after whatever problem we have and there was no waiting. And I wish it could all be done at a cost that we taxpayers can afford. Unfortunately, it was never quite that way and wishing for the old days will not get us there. We have hung on to these wishes for a long time and tried hard to get it to work for us today, but it is not happening. As we all know, change is happening, but it is not necessarily the kind of change we want.

I want you to know that all of the talk, all of the books and all of the pilot projects about health care have not gone to waste. With so many people trying so hard to get it to work it has encouraged me and I am very thankful that no one has given up.

IQSA *can* bring about good change. So, there you have it. The IQSA system does not recommend fewer doctors or nurses, does not recommend closure of hospitals or fewer beds, but even though these factors do not change, it will be difficult to move ahead. Opposition will still be there. What it does require is a change in mindset and that is by far the most difficult thing to change.

IQSA may also lessen future funding disputes between the provinces and the federal government. To speed up adoption of the system it might be helpful if the federal government would invest in the system by helping to fund development of trans provincial border health care. This could be accomplished by one simple rule. All patient care that requires crossing a provincial border for care would have additional funding provided by the federal government.

Have a great day and thank you for your time.

IQSA Health Care System
Implementation Timeline

(A very general example with many changes in consultation anticipated)

Year 1

Phase out family physician program. Offer training to family physicians to become specialist while they work. Train additional RNPs and build primary care clinics. Decide the types of care to be provided at each IQSA RR

Year 2

Train Paramedics to meet the need at primary emergency care centres. Build the centres.

Consult with IQSA RR to decide their focus (two or three specialties). Decide location of focused units within IQSA RR area. Calculate 24/7 staffing and bed requirements (i.e., 200-, 300-, or 400-bed unit) based on servicing the province with future expansion possibilities. Note: each IQSA RR will have one of each size of focused units.

Year 3

Design and build small consultation and coordination centre (H2C) at all Focused Centres of Excellence. Set out communication protocol. Train all FS to become VCS, include protocols for consultation. Rotate specialists for the H2C. Design the practice guidelines for standard care using an evidence-based model for use by the consultation specialist and focused specialists. Train all required health care providers in guidelines for communication with the H2C.

Year 4

Approve hospital minor renovation budget. and provide funding for Focused Centres of Excellence. Train nurses and other staff at tertiary care hospitals on the new protocols. Start with each IQSA RR area doing one specialization. Reconfigure existing beds to meet the need of a large unit. These are called Focused Centres of Excellence. Concentrate physician work. Design a streamline work process. Include a staff and physician communication protocol. The unit should be able to treat most patients within one to four days. ICU patients have no time limit. Afterward, the patient may be transferred to a tertiary care hospital. All hospitals without Focused Centres of Excellence will only provide tertiary service with virtual focused physicians.

Year 5

Design and renovate some ambulance stations to include multi-purpose room suitable for use as a transfer bus, terminal holding area. Train paramedics in suturing, ultrasound or x-ray use for long-bone fracture imaging, mini-laboratory use and advance skills in diagnosing and treating additional conditions.

Year 6

Arrange bus transfer service between cities for the first Focused Centre of Excellence. Gradually develop the transportation network as each IQSA RR develop their own Focused Centres of Excellence. Patients embarking or disembarking a bus at the transport terminals will use smaller vehicles to reach their destination in the local area.

Year 7

Renovate more hospitals to accommodate Focused Centres of Excellence.

Year 8

Set up medical tourism program with advertising in target countries. Provide additional staff training if required.

Year 9

Add additional focus units in each IQSA RR area repeating above steps for first focused unit.

Year 10

Develop medical tourist packages (i.e., transportation, hotel, surgery). Start bringing in medical tourists.

Year 11

Develop ancillary services at E-Stat centres if desired.

Acronyms and Terms

ACP (Advanced-Care Paramedic): ACP's staff the air ambulance helicopter.

E-Stat Centre: It is an acronym-based term meaning *E*mergency – *S*ervices, *T*reatment *A*nd *T*ransport. This is the name given to a multi-service centre. To be recognized as an E-Stat centre, it would provide primary emergency care by primary emergency care paramedics and an ambulance station staffed by paramedics. Optional services would include a medical transport terminal with holding room, a nurse practitioner clinic for primary care, an adult drop-in centre for routine patient monitoring, a fire first-response/rescue truck, a police sub-station or other services not yet identified. All services at the E-Stat would operate 24/7/365. If the right combination of services was included, these centres could become disaster response centres.

EMR: Electronic medical records.

FCoE (Focused Centres of Excellence): Large specialized units designed to service the entire province or a large area with focused physician specialists in attendance 24/7/365.

FS (Focused Specialists): Sometimes referred to as virtual focused specialists (VFS) These are the admitting/attending specialists at the Focused Centres of Excellence and provide hands-on and virtual care 24/7/365. These specialists will admit the patient and also attend the same patient for the full length of stay which includes their stay at tertiary hospitals, primary care centres, and primary emergency care centres. All virtual care is provided by video conferencing with patients and staff daily, or as required, and filing care plans and updates with the H2C.

H2C (Health Consultation Centre): The virtual consult specialist (VCS) may physically work from this location or virtually from anywhere. The centre will coordinate the care throughout the system, book a bed, and refer transport needs to the HTC as required.

HTC (Health Transport Centre): This centre coordinates the transport of patients throughout the province and manages the fleet of buses and other vehicles.

IQSA (Integrated, Quality, Sustainable, Accessible Health Care System): This is the system described in this book.

IQSA RR: This refers to Integrated, Quality, Sustainable, Accessible, Referral Region and are the IQSA equivalent to the old LHIN territory designation. Map 8 Ontario Local Health Integration Network 2015 www.150statscan.gc.ca/nl/pub/82-402-x/2017001/maps-cartes/rm-er08-eng.htm

LHIN (Local Health Integration Network) A local body created by the Ontario Ministry of Health and Long-Term Care to oversee local health care. They are no longer in existence but the area they covered is now designated as IQSA RR.

PA (Public Administration)

PC (Primary Care): This is where RNP and others work.

PCP (Primary Care Paramedic)

PEC (Primary Emergency Care): This is care that does not require admission to a hospital.

PECC (Primary Emergency Care Centre): A centre where primary emergency paramedics provide primary emergency care 24/7.

RNP (Registered Nurse Practitioner): Sometimes referred to as Nurse Practitioner or NP. The RNP provides care to the patients at a nurse practitioner-led primary care site. Other health care providers may also be found there.

Registered Paramedic Practitioner: A possible future designation for paramedics that provides care at a primary emergency care centre. The title would be obtained after graduating from a university undergraduate degree program that includes a one-year residency at a primary emergency care centre. Prior to the degree program being developed, paramedics with at least three years of experience would take additional training and complete a residency at a primary emergency care centre before becoming qualified.

Tertiary Hospital: A community hospital for the continuing care of patients after treatment at a Focused Centre of Excellence. They are staffed by nurses, other health care providers, and virtual focused physicians only. All emergency departments at these sites will remain open where they are, staffed by emergency physicians. It is here where emergency patients will be stabilized if required, before transport to a Focused Centre of Excellence if required.

Telehealth Ontario: Open 24/7 a nurse will provide advise or health information and tell you where to go for the care you need. They do not diagnose or provide medicine. The service is free.

VCS (Virtual Consult Specialist): Sometimes referred to as a consult specialist. A consultation specialist provides a second opinion which is always evidence based. They also provide a connection between health care providers and a focused specialist at the Focused Centre of Excellence. This connection occurs often between health care providers such as nurse practitioners, primary emergency care paramedics, registered nurses, physician specialists/family physicians, emergency physicians, and focused specialists. They do this without ever coming into physical contact with the patient.

VDT (Virtual Diagnostic Team): They assist in diagnosing difficult cases.

BIBLIOGRAPHY
(OPTIONAL READING)

American Journal of Public Health 2015 April, IIeana L. Pina, MD, MPH, Perry D. Cohen, PHD, David B, Larson, MD. MBA, Lucy N. Marion, RN, PHD, MN, Marion R. Sills, MD, MPH. Leif I. Solberg, MD, and Judy Zerzan, MD, MPH *A Framework for Describing Health Care Delivery Organizations and Systems*

Canadian Institute for Health Information Jan. 2007, *Analysis in Brief Understanding Emergency Department Wait Times: How Long Do People Spend in Emergency Departments in Ontario?*

Emergency Medical Services, Education Agenda for the Future: A SYSTEMS APPROACH, publish date unknown 1996? NHTSA The National Highway Traffic Safety Administration

HPRAC, Jan. 2009, *Critical Links, Transforming and Supporting Patient Care*, A Report to the Minister of Health and Long-Term Care on Mechanisms to Facilitate and Support Interprofessional Collaboration and a New Framework for the Prescribing and Use of Drugs by Non-Physician Regulated Health Professions.

Joshua Tepper, 1992-2001, Canadian Institute for Health Information, @ 2004 Canadian Institute for Health Information, *The Evolving Role of Canada's Family Physicians*

CBC Canadian Press Toronto Posted Dec. 04, 2019 *Nearly 70,000 patients harmed in Ontario's hospitals each year:* Auditor CBC News Auditor General Bonnie Lysyk (Paul Chiasson/Canadian Press)

Commission on the Future of Health Care Services: Discussion paper No. 17 *Delivering Health Care Services: Public, Not for Profit, or Private?* By Raisa B. Deber, Ph.D. University of Toronto

CBC Saskatchewan Daniella Ponticelli, *Expanding scope for pharmacists, paramedics, nurses on the table as Sask. Holds consultations*

About the Author

Born and raised in Northern Ontario I worked as a Paramedic for 37 years. During that time, I saw a slow but steady decline in health care beginning in the 1990's when hospitals were forced to close beds and then hospitals themselves closed. After all the layoffs, new nurses were hired as part time. It was often hard to find one in the hospital that could take a report because they were always short staffed. Physicians were restricted in their OR time to save money. This forced patients to wait a long time for surgery. Ambulance services were hard hit also. I experienced many changes in management taking us from public to private and eventually back to public. I was very fortunate to have been able to hang on to my job. Many did not. I must say however that during my career some things did improve, better training, better equipment more vehicles and staff but we still could not keep up to rising call volume. It was not unusual to get our 1200 lunch at 300 and work fourteen hours instead of twelve. Toward the end of my career, I found it very stressful and although I never went off on PTSD, I understood why it was happening. I think one of the things that bothered me the most was lining up in the hospital hallways, not able to get the patients the help they needed or respond to 911 calls. I knew if things were done a little differently it would not be this way. One thing that I think did help me was the fact that whenever I was stressed about something I would begin writing. I came up with many ideas that came to fruition and it gave me hope. Maybe this will be another.

Never stop believing it's possible.

Richard Powlesland

REFERENCES

i. Cameron MacLean Aug. 24, 2022, CBC News, *Up to 750 Manitobans could get hip, knee surgeries out of province under new agreements.*

ii. Roy J Romanow Q.C.Nov.2002 *Building on Values, Commission on The Future of Health Care in Canada*, Final Report,

iii. Bryan Thomas and Colleen Flood, Dec. 2015, Winnipeg Free Press, *Modernize Not Privatize Medicare* Evidence Network (https;//evidencenetwork.ca/tag/canada/)

iv. Ernie Stokes, managing director, Robin Somerville, director of corporate research services, Jan 15, 2008, the Centre for Spatial Economics (C4SE) *The Economic Cost of Wait Times in Canada* page 3 prepared by the Centre for Spatial Economics for the Canadian Medical Association.

v. Megan Knoedler April 20, 2017 Mayo Clinic Medical Science Blog *Economies of scale: volume in health care.*

vi. James B. Lieber 2015 OR Books https://www.jstor.org/stable/j. ctt18z4gww *Killer Care: How Medical Error Became America's third Largest Cause of Death, and What Can Be Done About It.* In the article he refers to a medical text in the field, Understanding Patient Safety by Robert M. Wachter, M.D., of the University of California Medical School at San Francisco.

vii. Dr. Howard Ovens, Kathy Stevenson, Wendy Cheung, David Dushenski, Dr. Jeff Eisen, Carolyn Farquharson, Jane Foster, Susan Harper, Joy McCarron, Dr. Naveed Mohammed. Dr. Tim Rutledge,

Roz Smith, Heather Stewart, Paula May Ponesse, OHA Bulletin Wed Dec.17, 2005 Medical Directives.

viii.   CBC News Sudbury June 05, 2017 *Ontario First nurse practitioner clinic marks 10 years since opening.*

ix.   Brian Goldman, 2013 CBC Radio, *White Coat, Black Art.*

x.   Callam Rodya, Nov. 19, 2008 Health Quality Ontario, CTV *News report paints grim picture.*

xi.   Alex McKeen Wed. April 7, 2022. The Star, Vancouver Bureau *Amid shortages of family doctors across Canada med school grads increasingly don't want the jobs*

xii.   Kristopher Morrison Jan 25, 2013 National Post Canada ERs without doctors? *New rural emergency centres rely on nurses and paramedics at night.*

xiii.   Martin Schuldhaus, summer 2011. Alberta College of Paramedics, *Paramedics Rely on Expanding Scope of Practice to Improve Rural Health Care.* Paramedics 20 issue 41

xiv.   Sophie Borland, Health Correspondent, Aug 15 2015 Daily Mail UK *The Paramedic Will See You Now: Staff with 16 weeks' training to stand in for GP's*

xv.   Dyrbye, Liselotte N. MD; Thomas, Mathew R. MD; Shanafelt, Tait D. MD April 2006 Academic Medicine Volume 81-Issue 4, p. 354-373 *Systematic Review of Depression, Anxiety, and Other Indicators of Psychological Distress Among US and Canadian Medical Students.*

xvi.   Haute Autorite de Sante HAS 2 Avenue du Stade de France-93218 Saint-Denis La Plaine Cedex, ANAP appui sante & medico-social April 2012 *Day Surgery : An Overview.*

xvii. John Dujay, news editor for Canadian HR Reporter, May 11 2020, Fraser Institute Study *Wait times cost economy more than $2 billion in 2019 study,*

xviii. Kenneth L. Davis Sept. 15, 2014, WSJ, *Hospital Mergers Can Lower Costs and Improve Medical Care*

xix. Jeremy Petch, PHD, Irfan A, Dhalla MD, David A Henry, MB, Susan E. Schultz, MA, MSC, Richard H. Glazier, MPH, MD, Sacha Bhatia, MBA, MD, Andreas Laupacis, MD, 2012, Data Matters [30] Healthcare Policy vol.8 No.22012 Public *Payments to Physicians in Ontario Adjusted for Overhead Costs.*

xx. Jacqueline LaPointe, Revcycle Intelligence, (https://revcycleintelligence.com.) Practice Management News, A 2016 Strategy&, created a report, (https://www.strategyand.pwc.com/reports/size-should-matter) *Key Strategies for Health Systems to Achieve Economies of Scale,* page 2/7

xxi. Pricewaterhousecoopers, May 2002, HealthCast Tactics, HealthCast 2010 Series, page 5, *A Blueprint for the Future.*

xxii. In a report by Pricewaterhousecoopers titled HealthCast Tactics, A Blueprint for the Future, May 2002, part of The HealthCast 2010 Series under the heading Creating the Future Hospital System page 12.

xxiii. Megan Ogilvie, Health reporter, Feb. 14, 2022, https://www.thestar.com/news/gta/2022/02/14/catastrophic-surgical -backlog-in-ontario-will-take-years-to-clear-doctors-say.html *Catastrophic surgical backlog in Ontario will take years to clear, doctors say.*

xxiv. County of Renfrew Ontario Canada, Dec.20,2022, *Point of Care Ultrasound Certification for Community Paramedics. Release Date, Dec 19 2022 Renfrew County Paramedics break new ground in Point of Care Ultrasound.*

xxv.   Lisa Priest, Toronto Star Reporter (The Saturday Star) Sept. 27,
1997, Atkinson Fellowship, *We're flying blind over tests on MD's*

xxvi. .OECD Sept. 2015 www.oecd.org/health page 8 *Fiscal Sustainability
of Health Systems, Bridging Health and Finance Perspectives.*

xxvii.   Jane Stevenson Mar. 12 2019, The Toronto Sun, by the Calgary
based think tank secondstreet.org *More Canadians are leaving the
country for health care: Report,* Statistics Canada, A policy brief titled
Flight of the Sick,

xxviii.   CTV News, Wed, April 14, 2010, Canadian Press, Analysis of
Health-care spending by the Toronto-based Dale Orr Economic
Insight, *Wide gaps in health spending across Canada.*

xxix. Katherine Fierlbeck, Dalhousie University, Commission on the
Future of Health Care in Canada, Discussion Paper NO. 15, August
2002, *Paying to Play? Government Financing and Health Care
Agenda Setting.*

xxx. KPMG Dec. 17, 2014, *Staying power – success stories in
global healthcare.*

xxxi. Abby Goodnough, Dec. 17, 2015 The New York Times, http://nyti.
ms/1Zf2tnY *Kaiser Permanente Plans Open a Medical School*